THE EMERGENCY MIND

ISBN: 9798746482327

Cover Design: Rachel Connors and Bridget Hilton, www.BridgetHilton.com

Book Design: Janis Dworkis, www.JanisDworkis.com, www.LaureateLifePress.com

www.EmergencyMind.com

Printed in the United States of America
First Printing 2021

Sangfroid Press
Los Angeles, CA

THE EMERGENCY MIND

Wiring Your Brain for Performance Under Pressure

Dan Dworkis, MD PhD FACEP

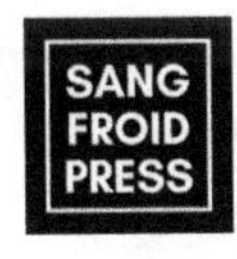

Los Angeles

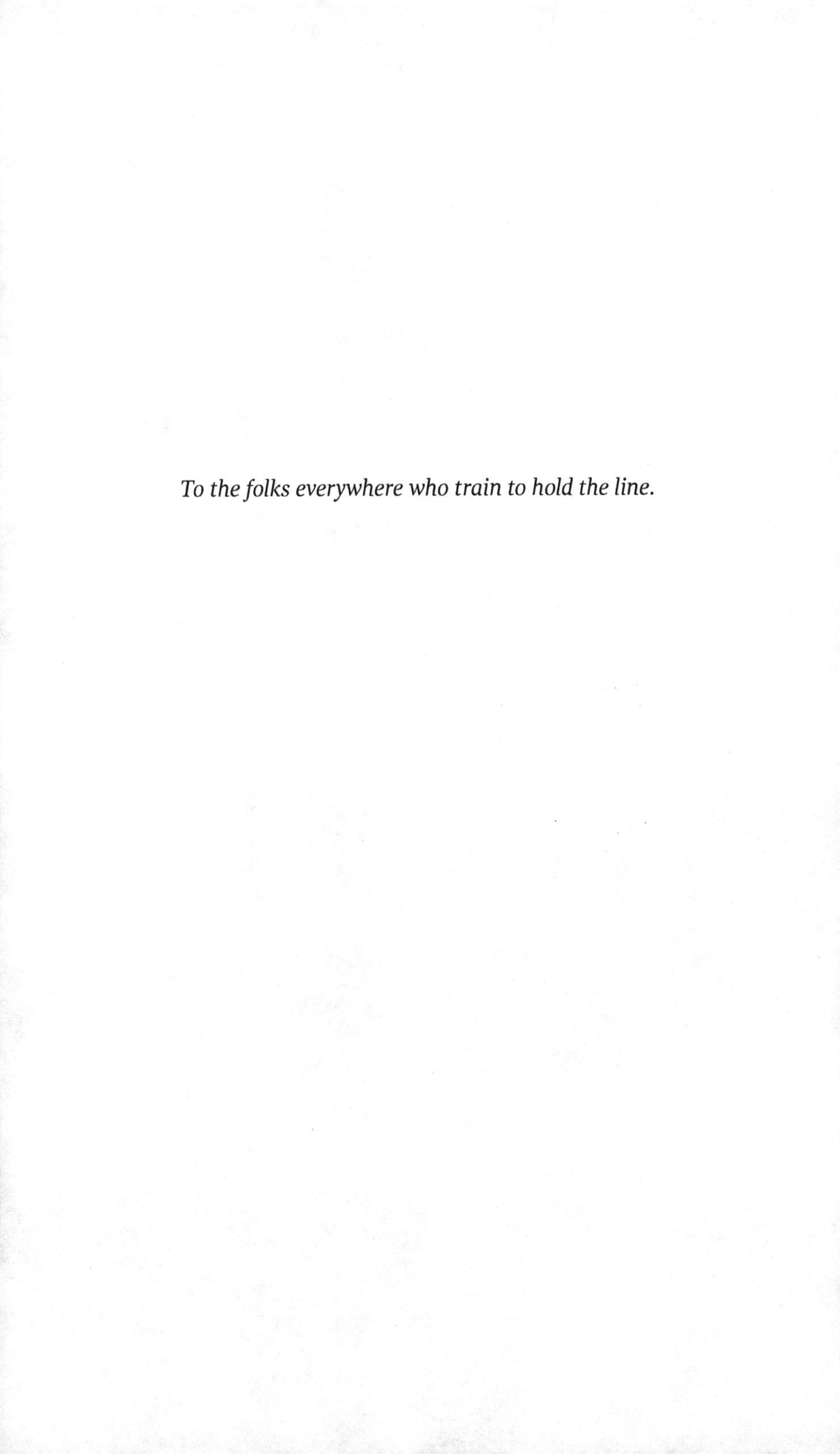

To the folks everywhere who train to hold the line.

The Emergency Mind:

(1) the "mental toolkit" you rely on when confronted
     by a crisis.

(2) the set of models, tools, and concepts used by
     skilled providers to successfully apply their
     knowledge under pressure.

CONTENTS

INTRODUCTION

During one of my first weeks in medical school, I found myself holding a young man's arm above his head to keep him from moving while an emergency doctor cut open his chest.

Like all first-year students, in addition to my lectures and sessions in the anatomy lab, I spent time shadowing experienced physicians as they did their work, watching and learning what it meant to be a doctor. While many of my classmates were assigned to pediatricians' offices or followed surgeons into operating rooms, I went down to the grit and wonderful chaos of the emergency department.

I was deeply happy and I was completely lost. I watched in wonder, and occasionally horror, as the various emergency teams went deftly from room to room treating patients who were screaming, crying, and bleeding. I watched them do their best to provide comfort, relieve suffering, and try to make a difference despite what seemed like total disaster swirling around them. How could they be so calm when everyone around them was anything but? Could I ever be like that?

It came to a head one day when an overhead alarm signaled the incoming ambulance that would bring that young man into the emergency department. One of the attending doctors pulled me into a trauma bay and told me to stand in the corner, put gloves and a mask on, and get ready. I had no idea what "get ready" meant—in fact, I did not even know where the mask was—but I nodded and got to it. Standing silently at the edge of the room, I saw for the first time what happens when trained experts spin themselves up and mentally prepare to try to save a life. I felt such awe at these people and at the transition they were going through right in front of me—such awe as they transformed from relaxed and joking to something else, something I had never seen before.

We heard the sirens approaching as the ambulance came in, and everyone in the room snapped to their positions. The paramedics rushed through the trauma doors with our patient on a gurney, and the first thing I noticed was how young he was—late teens, maybe twenty, just slightly younger than me. The second thing I noticed was the blood. He had been shot at least once in the chest and there was blood everywhere, just flowing out of him down the gurney and onto the ground.

As I kept watching, the emergency team slid him to the exam table and rapidly identified the most life-threatening of his injuries: a bullet had punctured his lung, and air was building up rapidly in his chest. As the doctors explained, unless they cut into his chest right then to make a hole for the air to escape and relieve the pressure, his heart might stop, and he might die.

The young man was panicked, bleeding, and confused, but the procedure had to happen immediately. One of the doctors turned to me and yelled the order to join and help. "You, med student, get in here and hold him down. Don't let him move that arm. Tell him it's going to be okay!"

So, I did. I stepped forward and held his arm down. I held his hand, looked him in the eyes, and told him he was going to be okay. I told him we were here for him, that we were going to do our best. Of course, I had no idea if he was going to be okay. I didn't even know what it meant to "do our best" in that situation. I just held on tight and told him I was there for him, that I would give him whatever little skill I had to offer.

Thankfully, all the other people in the room that night did know what to do. They had trained to be able to diagnose and treat his injuries. They had trained to cut through the mental fog I was experiencing as I saw the blood and felt the young man's fear. They had trained to bring their knowledge to bear in this kind of a chaotic situation in order to work to save a life.

So, they did. Nurses secured IV lines and administered pain medicine and warm fluids. The doctors successfully opened his chest and placed a chest tube to decompress the buildup of air. Clerks registered him, police officers took his statement, and a chaplain was on standby in case he wanted to talk. In the waiting room, peers from his community, who had also been through serious trauma, stood witness and talked his family through what would come next. I am sure there were many, many other aspects of that young man's care that went smoothly and well—things I was far too green to even have noticed at the time.

With the chest tube in place, the first critical moment had passed, and the team continued the resuscitation and examined him for other signs of trauma. He improved rapidly and was whisked away to the operating room to repair the injury to his lung. So far as I know, he recovered fully, and now leads a healthy (and, I hope, peaceful and happy) life.

The members of the emergency team debriefed and moved on to see their next patients, but I could not stop thinking about that young man and about the team taking care of him—a team with which I had participated so briefly and in such a small role. The gap between where I had been standing holding him and where those providers stood as they competently and compassionately treated him seemed impossibly large.

Intellectually though, I knew that gap could be crossed. Like me, every doctor in that room had started out at some point as a first-year medical student. I knew the skills I had witnessed—whatever it was that had allowed them to perform so well under pressure—must be skills that could be learned. They were skills I could learn, skills I knew I wanted to learn.

Over the fifteen or so years since that night—as I completed medical school, trained to become a board-certified emergency physician, and stepped into my role as attending faculty—I have often thought about that patient and the team I watched care for him. I have continued to think about the gap I felt so viscerally that day, and about what it takes to move from being an overwhelmed and occasionally terrified amateur to a calm and capable professional. Through training and practice, introspection and conversation, it became more and more clear to me that making this transition involves two distinct parts: first, you have to learn the medicine, and second you need to learn how to successfully apply that medical knowledge under pressure.

This book is not about the first part. It is not about learning medicine or gaining a deep knowledge of any particular craft. It won't help you choose an antibiotic or read an X-ray image, and it certainly does not contain medical advice. Instead, this book is about learning to work with the second part of the puzzle: it's about training to bring your skills to bear when the heat is on and wiring your brain to perform at your best during times of crisis.

I wrote this book because—as a practicing emergency physician and an assistant professor of emergency medicine—I am convinced this gap is crossable; I am convinced that wherever you are starting from as you read this, you can learn to apply knowledge under pressure. I wrote this book because I believe deeply that your ability to perform when it matters most depends directly on how you think, act, and train now, before an emergency strikes. Ultimately, I wrote it because I wish I'd had it when I went home that first day, and when I went home from so many shifts across the years trying to make sense of what I had seen and how I could improve my performance.

In the pages that follow, I lay out a series of mental models I have come to rely on when I practice and teach emergency medicine. These ideas describe the fundamentals of applying knowledge under pressure—concepts like handling uncertainty, accepting imperfection, and balancing structured and creative thinking. All these models have been proven in the rapidly changing and high-impact circumstances of the emergency department. They also have applications in your day-to-day life outside the hospital.

While the stories and examples in the book are primarily based in emergency medicine, you don't have to actively practice—or even want to practice—emergency medicine to benefit from their use. Whatever craft you want to master, these mental models will help you deploy your skills under suboptimal, stressful, or even adversarial conditions. Personally, I have found they are just as applicable to my study of jiu-jitsu, surfing, and navigating Los Angeles traffic as they are to emergency medicine.

You can read the models individually in the order they are presented or skip around and explore how they function in pairs or clusters. However you choose to approach them, remember that they function best with practice and frequent use. To get the most out of these mental models, you need to test them, experiment with them, modify them, and make them your own. They are presented here not as gospel or as the only way to do things, but in the spirit of martial arts legend Bruce Lee, who famously said that you should, "Absorb what is useful. Reject what is useless. Add what is essentially your own."

As you start to make your way across that gap between amateur and professional—as you learn to build your emergency mind and wire your brain for performance under pressure—it is my hope that this book will serve you as a guide. When you have built your skills to the point that you've found better models, come teach me, and we can test them together.

From one student of human performance under pressure to another, I hope you enjoy.

Dan Dworkis, MD PhD FACEP
Los Angeles, CA
May 2021

WHAT IS AN EMERGENCY?

Imagine you're the doctor in charge during a busy shift at a high-volume emergency department. Everything is running along smoothly and you're working with a patient with abdominal pain, when one of the most experienced nurses runs up to you looking concerned. There was a high-speed, multiple-vehicle accident on the highway nearby, and in the next few minutes several seriously injured individuals will arrive all at once. As you walk out of the room, you hear the sirens approaching. Everything in the department seems to grind to a halt as all eyes focus on you. How would you react? What would you do to ensure that you—and your team—perform at your best during this crisis?

Unless you had trained extensively in providing emergency care, advanced trauma life-support protocols, and interdisciplinary team management, chances are you would struggle to perform up to your potential. In fact, even if you've already completed medical school—if you have medical training and knowledge on paper—you would probably still find it difficult to actually bring your skills to bear under this kind of pressure.

Of course, you would be in good company. Almost everyone would struggle in this type of crisis. If you take a group of individuals early in their medical training and ask them how they responded to their first real emergency, you would likely hear, "I knew what to do in theory, but I just froze." Or, perhaps, "I wanted so much to help but I just couldn't move." However, if you ask a group of experienced emergency providers about their performance after a difficult crisis, you tend to hear things like: "That was challenging, but we were able to bring all the resources we had online and perform at a high level." Or they might say, "I relied on my training and pressed forward despite the circumstances and I'm proud of my team's performance."

How do providers get to the point where they can make those types of statements? How can you?

The good news is that no one is born this way. The ability to move past your fear and confusion, organize a team around a goal, and mount an effective response to that multi-victim accident is not an innate gift. Instead, performing under pressure is a set of skills that can be broken down, trained, and put back together again.

This book is about choosing to train those skills, about choosing to train to respond to an emergency. It won't teach you how to put in a chest tube or splint a broken bone, but it will help you apply every piece of knowledge you have under whatever circumstances you face. While you cannot control what emergencies come your way, you do control how you prepare; you control what you do now to build your emergency mind and wire your brain to perform under pressure.

So, what is an emergency? Clearly, this incoming multi-victim trauma is an emergency, or, more accurately, a group or series of emergencies. People's lives are on the line, resources will be stretched thin, crucial decisions will need to be made correctly and rapidly. The situation is fluid and likely to change quickly, requiring improvisation and permitting you minimal time to study the problem before you are forced to act. While you and your team might have prepared for similar scenarios, it is very unlikely that you ever would have practiced in this exact set of circumstances.

Of course, you don't have to be an emergency provider or work in a hospital to face emergencies. Situations where everything is on the line and how you perform makes the difference between success and failure happen often in the military and law enforcement, firefighting, and the airline industry. They also are common occurrences in sport and business. In fact, you may face elements of an emergency situation anytime you need to make good choices in tight time frames when emotions are running high or the pressure is on. Perhaps you're trying to meet a critical deadline at work while helping a sick family member at home. Maybe you find yourself confronted by a dangerous aggressor in the parking lot when leaving a store, or you need to make a split-second decision when a drunken driver swerves into your lane on the highway.

In or out of the emergency department, all emergencies share three common structural characteristics:

- Emergencies involve uncertainty.
- Emergencies have high-impact outcomes.
- Emergencies occur under significant pressure.[1]

Uncertainty describes the lack of clear and unequivocal knowledge about the problem you face, what choices you should make, or both. Medical emergencies start with high levels of uncertainty when the patient has just arrived at the emergency department, since the details of what's happening or the extent of their illness or injuries is usually unclear. During the course of diagnosing and treating the patient, your uncertainty typically diminishes as you build a coherent model of the cause of their suffering and identify what you can do to help. Alternatively, your level of uncertainty might spike unpredictably as their condition changes rapidly or if they begin to decompensate.

Interestingly, during a cardiac arrest, uncertainty is sometimes less a factor than at other points: you still might not know the reason for the cardiac arrest, but you know very well what steps you need to take to treat it. In this case, there are well-studied algorithms like the advanced cardiac life support protocol that you can begin to implement even when you don't yet know the underlying cause of the problem. Recognizing local high and low points in the uncertainty of a case, as well as discontinuities in the pairing between uncertainty around cause and uncertainty around response, are crucial skills in operating under pressure.

While uncertainty can never be fully eliminated, it can sometimes be reduced by trading time or resources for more certainty. In the emergency department, you gain certainty on a patient's situation by performing lab tests, physical exams, and imaging, or by attempting a particular treatment and seeing the results. You might also use the "test of time" and perform serial observations on an undifferentiated patient to gain more certainty as their course progresses.

Outside the emergency department, you similarly seek to reduce uncertainty during a crisis by performing tests and updating your beliefs about the emergency you face. For example, if a driver is swerving into your lane, you usually respond by rapidly looking to either side to clarify your position and identify options for a potential response.

Impact describes the gravity or severity of the potential outcomes of the situation. In an emergency, the potential impact is always high. A patient brought to the emergency department suffering a heart attack is in a high-impact scenario, as is a child with severe asthma who presents barely able to breathe. In each case, the threat of significant injury or even death is real, obvious, and typically weighs heavily in both the minds of the patient and the treating team. Outside of the emergency department, a family waking up to a house fire would certainly be in a high-impact scenario, as would the captain of a ship that had drifted off course and was rapidly approaching another vessel.

While the impact of an emergency might not be known specifically, the perception of the possible impact is just as important an influence on your performance. In an extremely personal example of this, I was once a patient in a small hospital in India when I found an air bubble in my intravenous line. Knowing what I do now, I can say the bubble was small enough to likely have had little to no actual impact on me. But at the time—before my medical training—I was convinced it was going to kill me. I was terrified and, responding to my perception of the potential impact, I quickly turned off the IV drip. Thankfully, the nurse kept me from ripping it out entirely and then explained the situation.

The potential impact of a situation almost always feels larger from the inside than it does from the outside. This is immediately obvious to anyone who has ever had "minor" surgery. As decision expert and former professional poker player Annie Duke talks about in her book *Thinking in Bets*, gaining accurate "outside view" information on our situation is crucial to mitigate the sometimes disproportionate "inside view" effects of a personally significant potential impact.[2]

Whatever the potential impact of a situation is, fear of this impact can lead to paralysis; you can find yourself unable to make a decision because you are so preoccupied with what the impact might be. Of course, not making a decision is, in and of itself, a decision. As we will explore throughout the mental models in this book, coming to terms with potentially difficult outcomes is part of your job when you want to perform better during a crisis. Handling your fear and pressing forward anyway is always a better answer than paralysis.

Pressure describes the mix of internal and external factors that can create the suboptimal conditions in which you will respond to the emergency. The most common form of pressure during an emergency is time pressure; rarely, if ever, will you have all the time you want to make a decision during a crisis. Managing the flow of decision making under time pressure is a core ability for emergency providers. It spans resource allocation, utilizing intelligent decision aids, and optimization of the stress response, among a wide variety of other skills. Multiple mental models in subsequent chapters explore this issue in depth.

Aside from time pressure, emergencies often involve circumstances that are extremely challenging emotionally. You may face pressure from your own experience of suffering or from watching other people suffer. If you or someone close to you is involved directly in the crisis, you might feel emotions like fear, anger, or sadness. If the situation is somewhat more abstract for you, crises may bring up intense feelings of compassion, empathy, or the desire to help others.

While these emotions can be powerful motivators to generate rapid and competent action, if improperly harnessed they can cloud your judgment and decrease your effectiveness. Emergency doctors who are parents, for example, often talk about the extra burden of fear they face when treating a sick child who reminds them of their own. Similarly, outside the emergency department, a pilot having to skillfully land a damaged plane might simultaneously have to handle the pressure of thinking about how her family would survive if she perished.

Your physiological readiness to handle complex loads also influences the pressure you experience during a crisis. Low stocks of internal resources such as nutrition, hydration, sleep, and recovery negatively affect performance and increase the pressure you feel. External factors like temperature, noise, or light conditions may also play a role in diverting your attention and increasing your cognitive load.[3]

Importantly, you typically feel pressure relative to your available resources, not on absolute scale. Maximizing your available resources before and during a crisis, and improving the efficiency of their use, can therefore reduce your perceived pressure. For example, if you were given ten seconds to cut through a rope, you would feel much more pressure if you had a butter knife than if you had a sharp razor blade. Accordingly, several of the mental models we explore in this book work both with reducing sources of pressure and improving resource availability.

While uncertainty, impact, and pressure are presented here as unique and separate structural components of an emergency, in practice they often blur into one another, causing confusion and negative synergy. For example, situations with significant levels of uncertainty and pressure—such as estimating if your car will fit into a particular parking space while others around you are honking their horns and yelling—can sometimes take on the feel of an impact much larger than what is actually involved. Maintaining an honest appraisal of the levels of these factors present in a situation can alert you to opportunities to improve your training and ability to perform during crises.

In addition to these three structural factors, all emergencies also involve a fourth component—the need to make decisions. Sometimes these decisions are large and external, such as how to deploy your limited resources when you're about to lead the resuscitation team in preparation for that incoming multi-casualty accident. Other times, the decisions are internal, such as how you choose to respond to an aggressive co-worker or an emotionally charged argument with a loved one. Regardless of the type of decision involved, decision making under pressure is a skill you can train, improve, and work to master.

To address the uncertainty, impact, and pressure you'll face in emergencies, and to improve your decision-making abilities, this book presents a series of the fundamental mental models used in emergency medical care and when responding to crises. These models are the core concepts that make up emergency providers' understanding of how physiology, decision making, systems design, and more combine to impact individual and team performance under stress.

To be useful, these mental models need to be explored and worked with, much in the way that raw clay needs to be worked and shaped before it can be used as a cup or a jar. The prescription of this book, therefore, is to understand and practice these mental models not just when you find yourself in an active emergency situation, but now, today, in your everyday life. In this way, when you do find yourself in a emergency—and you will—you will have the training you need to put these mental models to work and successfully deploy your knowledge when it counts most.

EMERGENCY MENTAL MODELS

Mental models are the conceptual frameworks we all use to explain how parts of reality work. Anytime you extrapolate information from sets of experiences to guide future actions, generate rules for how things are supposed to work, or balance sets of competing principles to fine tune a decision, you are using mental models to explore, map, and predict the world around and within you.[1]

Some mental models are simple but powerful ideas, like the concept of leverage, an intuitive concept with which you probably have a considerable amount of direct experience. Understanding leverage helps you explain why effort exerted in some places yields significantly different results than effort exerted in others. Used effectively, this mental model can guide you to more efficiently distribute your energy so that small actions can lead to disproportionately large effects.

Other mental models are more complicated: they may involve multiple components which interact in complex or non-intuitive ways, or they may represent parts of reality with which you do not have direct experience. Exploring and mastering these more complicated models can extend your reach beyond your personal experience and help you understand a diverse array of messy, real-life situations. For example, the Frank-Starling law is a mental model that describes how much blood the human heart will typically pump as a function of the volume of blood delivered to it.[2]

Generally speaking, the model states that the heart will match its output to its input across a wide array of physiologic states. Working with the Frank-Starling model helps you understand many aspects of cardiac physiology in both healthy and unhealthy hearts. You might never run physiological experiments yourself to validate the Frank-Starling curve, but you can leverage the model to help guide you in deciding optimal fluid resuscitation techniques or pharmacotherapy options for certain sick patients such as those with heart failure or cardiogenic shock.

Some mental models are unique to a particular field, while others cross over to multiple disciplines. For example, designing safer airbags in cars and making a new multi-vitamin both require understanding mental models about human anatomy and physiology. In one case, you would combine these models with fundamental concepts from physics, engineering, and materials science. In the other, you would add in mental models from biochemistry, pharmacology, and nutrition.

Like all theoretical constructs, mental models are imperfect but useful representations of reality. Each model has its own strengths and weaknesses and performs better at describing some parts of reality than others. While each mental model stands on its own, they are stronger and more useful when applied in combinations to emergency situations.[3] The ways in which they fit together, augment each other, and occasionally contradict one another are sometimes predictable and sometimes surprising depending on the context in which they are deployed.

The mental models in this book are used by individuals and teams practicing emergency medicine and delivering medical care in high-stakes environments that are full of uncertainty and involve significant pressure. They are just as applicable outside of the emergency department as they are inside. That said, all mental models are tuned to a specific use case, and these tend to become more powerful and accurate as situations become more dire.

It's important to note that the mental models in and of themselves will not help a sick patient or ensure that you perform well under pressure any more than the idea of compound interest will, in and of itself, make you wealthy. To wire your brain to perform under pressure—to make sure you can employ these models when you need them in a pinch—these ideas must be practiced, modified to suit your individual needs, and then applied again and again both inside and outside of crisis situations.

The twenty-five mental models described here comprise a core subset of the many, many models that you might harness to respond effectively when you need to apply your skills during an emergency. They are presented here in five groups:

I Applying Knowledge Under Pressure

II Handling Uncertainty and Imperfection

III Making Critical Decisions

IV Building from Core Values

V Balancing Competing Forces

The first group, **Applying Knowledge Under Pressure**, contains models addressing the application of existing stores of knowledge under adverse conditions. These models include methods of mitigating the effects of stress and developing improved responses to impending disaster. The models in this group are deployed nearly constantly in the emergency department but become especially important during the most critical and chaotic cases when the barriers to deploying existing knowledge successfully become particularly high.

The second group, **Handling Uncertainty and Imperfection**, contains models that help you address gaps in your knowledge of the universe and complications in your decision making. Inherent in these models are ideas involving the limits of human understanding and performance, and the importance of expecting and planning for a certain degree of failure during a crisis. These models are useful when deployed either before or during an emergency and they can help you design and utilize structures that support "good" responses to "bad" outcomes.

The third group, **Making Critical Decisions**, contains models highlighting how to best make high- and low-impact decisions under significant pressure. The mental models in this group are used routinely by individuals and teams in emergency medicine to make better and faster decisions during complex cases. They will help you look several moves ahead to identify and address problems before they arise. While these models are primarily deployed while a crisis is already underway, your ability to use them depends on the work you put into them prior to an emergency situation.

The fourth group, **Building from Core Values**, contains models describing how to link the deepest beliefs you and your teammates hold to the cutting edge of your response during a crisis. These models explore how understanding your core values—for example, the commitment to do no harm—can shape the way you perform under pressure. Since these values are the foundation on which multiple aspects of your training and practice rely, formalizing and developing these structures early can pay dividends across both emergency and routine scenarios.

Finally, the fifth group, **Balancing Competing Forces**, contains models exploring the tension and trade-offs between pairs of often diverging goals that can occur during emergencies. These models describe the balance that is required when you try to solve critical problems with multiple inherent priorities and no perfect solution. They can be deployed prior to an event to help build intelligent systems and flexible teams, or during an event to help you rapidly make complex choices under pressure.

The boundaries of these five groups should be seen as very permeable and should serve as guidelines rather than strict dogma. Bringing models together across groups in alternative combinations will likely give rise to other important themes in emergency performance. Just as experimentation is necessary in the use of single models, you will need to practice connecting them in multiple ways and explore for yourself how the models can interreact and combine to improve performance under pressure.

NOTES ON PATIENT DETAILS
AND TERMINOLOGY

Throughout this book, I use examples of patient cases to illustrate concepts and explore how a mental model applies to real emergency situations. In the vast majority of instances, these cases are composites drawn together from the details of many individual patients to better convey a particular point. In the few instances when the details do come primarily from one single patient case, multiple facets of the case have been changed to preserve patient anonymity.

In the United States, care is often taken to distinguish between an emergency room and an emergency department. Where an emergency room is a single location for urgent medical care, an emergency department represents a larger and more complex entity with a dedicated medical staff and a greater array of activities and services. Additionally, the terminology used to describe an individual delivering emergency care can be divisive, and occasionally heated debate surrounds the use of the generic term "emergency provider."

The mission of this book is to provide information to everyone who performs under pressure, regardless of their circumstances. So, I have chosen to ignore these distinctions and use these terms fluidly and interchangeably. That said, since personally I am a physician who works in an emergency department, I will often default to that configuration for ease and clarity.

Maybe you provide care in an emergency department, a casualty ward, or an A&E. Maybe you work in a single room in a small clinic, in a tent in a field hospital, in the back of a helicopter, or simply on whatever surface you can find. Maybe you call yourself a provider, a physician, a nurse, an APP, or a student. Maybe you're an operator, a medic, a first responder, or something else entirely.

Whatever your title and wherever you practice, if you need to perform under pressure, this book is for you.

—D.D.

I

APPLYING KNOWLEDGE
UNDER PRESSURE

01

FIND THE CALM IN THE STORM

Where beginners see only chaos, experienced emergency providers are able to see the underlying "rhythm" in a crisis and identify time to think and act in even the worst situations. Finding these moments of calm during a crisis allows you the space to analyze your progress and pivot your response to more productive directions. When calm moments do not naturally occur, experts can use focused training and well-designed systems to create them.

I doubt I will ever forget the first cardiac arrest case I ran as the team leader. It was early in my residency training, and small details of the young woman's story are burned into my mind, crystal clear and superimposed on a background blur of frenzied activity. The first time you lead a team working a cardiac arrest like this often seems like running a full-bore sprint. Your patient's heart has stopped, and you might feel like you must therefore move as fast as possible.

Junior-level responses to emergencies like a cardiac arrest are often chaotic, disorganized, and centered around trying to simply move faster in every direction all at once. Inexperienced leaders pace aimlessly while yelling orders to everyone indiscriminately or mumbling them to no one. They micromanage the small decisions while losing sight of the big ones, and try to overpower the uncertainty and pressure by simply "grinding through" the problem.

Experienced emergency providers run a cardiac arrest case entirely differently. With practice, your thoughts and actions become centered on rhythm and flow over raw speed and force. Your strategies are built not on taking more actions, but on slowing down to identify and then execute only the best possible actions for that patient in that moment.

To accomplish this, the best leaders actively seek out and build moments of calm into even the most chaotic and critical cases. These "spare moments" allow you the time and space to improve decision making, process new information, and pivot to new directions. As a result, teams led by expert providers are focused, agile, and more effective at providing high-quality care.

In order to further explore how moments of calm bring a crucial advantage to experienced teams, let's break down one of the fundamental tools that emergency teams use to respond to a cardiac arrest—the advanced cardiac life support (ACLS) algorithms. These algorithms form the framework of optimal resuscitation during cardiac arrests of all types. They are deceptively simple on paper, yet there are vast differences between how skilled and unskilled teams run these algorithms in their attempts to diagnose and treat the causes of cardiac arrest.

Regardless of why a patient has suffered a cardiac arrest, you run ACLS in two-minute, highly organized cycles of cardiopulmonary resuscitation (CPR). Between each cycle, you briefly pause CPR to scan and identify the electrical rhythm of the patient's heart and assess for the return of a pulse.

This pause allows you to see if your actions up to this point fixed the problem and restarted your patient's heart. If not, you need to rapidly determine what you need to do differently next. Ideally, this pause lasts only a few seconds, because every moment you're pausing to analyze and decide is a moment your patient is not receiving CPR.[1]

During each two-minute round of CPR, you and your team also have a number of tasks to perform. You may decide to deliver medications or electrical shocks or perform procedures like obtaining intravenous access or placing a breathing tube. Alternatively, you may reach out to next of kin to involve them in decision making around end-of-life care. During the same two minutes, you must also observe and reflect on what is happening, work together to update your mental model of the patient's disease process, and make a plan that prioritizes future actions for the next two-minute cycle.

This is a lot of work to accomplish, especially if you are in "full sprint" or panic mode throughout the cycles. Carving out calmer spaces to think, process, and plan allows you and your team to absorb new information and provide better care during the next cycle. This differential advantage is particularly salient when you need to pivot to respond to a significant change in the patient's status, or when the initial treatments are not yielding the desired results and creative alternatives need to be considered.

Logistically, capitalizing on calm moments in the midst of complex emergencies involves identifying existing moments of calm during a case and purposefully training to generate new ones.

When I first started leading resuscitation teams, identifying existing moments of calm during an active cardiac arrest seemed impossible. But as skills evolve and your knowledge base deepens, it becomes easier and easier. The more expertise you develop in an area, the lower the mental costs of making individual decisions.[2]

Functionally, this decrease in the amount of time required to make high-quality decisions means that you will have more time available for other needs. With practice, you can reframe this extra time as "moments of calm" and train yourself to identify the moments that already exist between decisions. These bits of time become spaces in which you can think and recover—much in the same way that expert athletes train to utilize time between plays for reset and reflection.

Of course, since the amount of this "interstitial" time you have during a crisis is directly related to your expertise, novice providers have more difficulty anticipating, identifying, and using these moments. Understanding when the clouds typically part for more senior practitioners may generate cues for where and when more junior providers can look for calm moments, even if they don't inherently feel them yet themselves.

In parallel to identifying naturally occurring moments which lend themselves to calmer decision making, you can also proactively train yourself to generate moments of calm by removing extraneous cognitive load and offloading non-critical decision making. Environmental factors like heat or cold, internal factors like hunger or thirst, and external sources of noise or distraction all represent sources of extraneous cognitive load and take mental energy away from addressing the task at hand.

Wherever possible, addressing and minimizing these factors increases the resources you have available to perform your core work during an emergency. As a crucial example, knowing your teammates names, their training, and their preferred roles ahead of time reduces friction and improves teamwork. A corollary to this is that junior or new members of a team should always try to introduce themselves before a crisis strikes. Efficient work means more "leftover" time, which translates to more moments of calm.

Similarly, rapidly identifying decisions that do not need to be made in a particular moment leaves more mental energy available for the decisions that *do* need to be made. Automating certain processes—like by-default activating appropriate intensive care staff when a patient arrives in the emergency department in cardiac arrest—removes the need for some decisions. So do external decision-support aids—such as emergency action cards or wall charts that list doses of critical drugs—and proactively restricting communication to only that which is most essential.[3] As is the case with decreasing extraneous cognitive load, actively limiting lower-yield decision making leaves more time for moments of calm during the crisis. For example, questions about diet orders for other patients should not be brought up to a clinician who is actively coding a patient.

Finding calm in the midst of chaos is not easy, but it is something you can work to improve. To paraphrase the Stoic philosopher and Roman emperor Marcus Aurelius, "The closer a person is to calm, the closer they are to strength."[4] It is only by starting to look for and use moments of calm during a crisis that you will find this source of strength. So, the next time you find yourself in a tense but non-emergency situation, look for and attempt to generate moments of calm. Afterward, reflect on the resulting experience. You likely will be surprised how situations that initially feel like chaotic sprints actually have an underlying rhythm and natural spaces to think.

Take Action

Using moments of calm to regroup or pivot requires first identifying these moments in the middle of emergencies. If you already have expertise in an area, reflect on when you might feel the potential for a pause. Start to look for times that have lower levels of cognitive load or when you typically already find yourself taking a breath.

The next time you feel one of these moments, identify the pause to yourself either mentally or out loud, and try to actively analyze your position and plan your next move. The first several times you try this, you may only get as far as identifying the calm moment before your cognitive load again increases and you are swept into the next task—but even that is progress.

If you are more junior, consider asking more experienced operators when they're the calmest and when they're the most activated in a particular process. Even if you don't yet feel the calm yourself, looking for it where you're likely to find it will be helpful. For example, an emergency team might leave the trauma bay for thirty seconds while a patient is being X-rayed as part of an initial workup—an opportunity for experienced providers to regroup. Knowing this, a more junior provider might start to practice calming strategies during that exact moment.

If some repeating parts of an emergency are predictably the most chaotic—like the first few moments of a cardiac arrest—you can design simulation or mental visualization training to actively address these critical moments. Training like this can help decrease decision-making costs and free up energy for finding calm moments.

Alternatively, you might choose to train personal cues that remind you to look for calm moments. These could include taking your own pulse at the beginning of a critical case or taking two deep breaths while the paramedics are wheeling the patient into the room. Practicing these cues and developing the habit of looking for moments of calm outside of acute crises makes these tools more accessible to you during emergencies.

See Also

10 | Make "Plan B" Part of the Plan
20 | Rapidly Accept Reality
22 | Find Your Locus of Control

02

BECOME A STUDENT OF SANGFROID

Sangfroid—translated literally as "coldblooded"—is the ability to be calm under significant pressure. While it might seem like sangfroid is an innate talent only a few possess, it actually is a skill that anyone, including you, can develop. Time spent working on your craft is necessary but not sufficient to develop this ability. Mastering sangfroid requires deliberate practice involving experimentation and dedicated training under pressure.

Standing in the middle of a crowd of frenzied bystanders, a senior paramedic calmly holds pressure on a bleeding wound while marshaling her team and reassuring her patient. Synthesizing flows of incoming data to coordinate the efforts of multiple squads around him, an experienced fire captain coolly and effectively directs resources to respond to a building fire with multiple casualties. Unfazed by the dropping oxygen saturation and chirping alarms, an emergency doctor transitions smoothly to her backup plan when her primary approach to placing a breathing tube fails and successfully saves her patient's life.

The ability of expert providers to stay calm and deploy their knowledge in chaotic environments is called "sangfroid," an amalgamation of the French words for blood (*sang*) and cold (*froid*). Literally meaning "cold-blooded," sangfroid is the skill of remaining cool and collected under pressure and performing at high levels of expertise during situations that involve significant stress or danger.

If you want to perform under pressure, you need to develop sangfroid. Without sangfroid, individuals operating under high loads of stress can freeze and panic, and teams working in rapidly changing or antagonistic environments may quickly fall apart. With sangfroid, you will bring calm, poise, and skill into the middle of disasters, and your performance under pressure will serve as an anchor that less skilled providers can rely on in the face of stress and danger.

While the gap between where you start and where you want to be with sangfroid might initially be large, sangfroid is a skill that anyone can learn through dedicated, specific training. To start with, it's important to dispel two common myths about where sangfroid comes from. Both of these myths were prevalent when I started consciously working to develop this skill, and chances are that you've heard some version of them, too.

First, sangfroid is not a fixed personality trait that you either have or you don't. The first time I interacted with a patient in medical school, I was a total mess—nervous, sweaty, and stumbling over my own name. Hardly what one would consider having sangfroid. With time and training though, I learned to observe my own reaction to stress and incrementally improve my ability to perform under pressure, slowly building my own sense of sangfroid.

Among emergency physicians, this story is hardly unique. Even providers who now show the most skill at handling pressure can relate stories of earlier versions of themselves struggling with sangfroid. As far as I have seen, no one is born with the ability to perform under pressure, it must be learned through training. So, even if you do not currently view yourself as a paragon of calm performance, knowing that sangfroid is a skill and not an innate character trait gives you the mental space to believe that you can improve.

Second, while deep experience in a field makes sangfroid easier to develop, sangfroid does not develop passively as a byproduct of training other skills. Put slightly differently, time spent mastering your craft is necessary but not sufficient to develop sangfroid. Conscious, deliberate training that is explicitly focused on high-pressure performance is required.

If building sangfroid were to happen passively as you train other skills, then the oldest people in the room—those with the most time spent training—would always be the coolest under pressure. Instead, it is the people and teams who specifically practice sangfroid who perform the best during a crisis.

For example, during a cardiac arrest, would you prefer to have a senior dermatologist or a much more junior emergency doctor lead the team providing life-saving care? While the dermatologist would have spent years studying medicine and mastering dermatology, the emergency doctor's training would have included deploying basic lifesaving skills in rapidly changing environments. Personally, I would pick the junior emergency doctor every time. You cannot assume that the dermatologist would have simply "picked up" how to handle an emergency along with studying dermatology any more than you would expect that lifting weights with your legs would significantly improve the strength of your upper body. Instead, if you want to perform at your highest level during emergencies, then you need to specifically train sangfroid as its own skill.

So, if sangfroid is not innate and it does not come as a byproduct from time spent working on your craft in general, how do you train sangfroid? The answer is you train it as you would any other skill: purposeful practice and experimentation. In other words, as you build your emergency mind, you must commit to become a student of sangfroid.

The first step in training sangfroid is to develop a sense of how you currently respond to pressure. Think of this like taking a placement test when you start to study a foreign language, or the first few days of running drills when you join a new team. Before you can design a training program for any particular skill, you need to assess your starting point.

When you get into tough situations, how do you tend to respond? Do you have certain habitual responses, specific things you tend to say or do? Some of these might be productive, like taking a deep breath and focusing on your next move. Others, like starting to yell or blame your team or your equipment, might be less productive or even detrimental. What about your internal environment? When faced with difficult situations do you get nauseated or short of breath? What does pressure feel like to you?

Not all of your answers to these questions are going to be pleasant, but as much as possible, try to answer honestly and in granular detail. The more you understand how you currently respond, the better your training will be later on.

Second, identify different models for more effectively responding to pressure. Some of these models might be small iterations on actions you're already taking. For example, you could take three deep breaths for three counts each, instead of just any deep breath. Perhaps you could modify the tone of your voice or practice saying slightly different words when you address your team. Alternatively, these different models might include ideas you've never tried before, or methods you see working for other people when you observe them under pressure.

Again, the more detail you capture with each of these models, the better. When starting to consider techniques that are very far from what you currently do, try to identify small steps or subprocesses that can bridge you from what you do now to what you want to attempt. For example, if you observe someone skilled at sangfroid who practices a full hour of yoga before each shift to generate a stress buffer, consider subgoals such as practicing yoga for 10 minutes before your shift.[1]

The third and most important step in developing skill at sangfroid is experimentation. You have to consciously practice different techniques of performance under pressure to find what works best for you. There are no substitutes and no shortcuts for this experimentation. In each experiment, your hypothesis will be trying or refining a method of responding to pressure. Your result will be the comparison of your external performance and your "feel" of your internal environment to what you identified in the first step as your current state of responding to pressure. As you improve, so will your benchmark of how you currently respond. Perfect mastery is not the goal; continued study and improvement is.[2]

One important note: The process of developing sangfroid is not at all linear and comparing your progress to that of others after a set amount of time might set you up for disappointment or failure. Milestones in structured training are of course important, but sangfroid is intensely personal; at its core, it is about who you are and how you relate to the universe. No one can teach you sangfroid, it is up to you to choose to study it.

Take Action

As described above, start with a fearless analysis of how you currently respond in difficult circumstances. Asking teammates or close friends to help you with this analysis, or to proactively watch you next time you are under stress can yield interesting, important, and sometimes uncomfortable results you might not otherwise be able to access.

When you're ready to begin experimenting, don't start in ultra-high pressure, life-or-death situations. Instead, start the experiments when you feel pressure during your everyday life—maybe when someone cuts you off in traffic and you have to swerve to avoid an accident, or you encounter an aggressive individual at work.

Logistically, it can help to be very explicit with your experiment. You might write down your intended actions and design formal experiments, such as: "When I feel pressure, I will take a breath, pause, and then physically move toward the problem." Alternatively, you could consider stating out loud to your team what you are trying and ask for feedback on whether or not it seemed to work. If your experiment works well, great; you can keep trying it during future challenges. If it does not, no problem, you can try another tactic.

With time and training, these small experiments will help you build a vision of what works for you personally. Each time you find something that works, you can keep applying it in situations with increasing amounts of pressure until you find yourself armed with a set of proven tools to face even extreme emergencies with calm and skill.

See Also

01 | Find the Calm in the Storm
06 | Practice *Wabi-Sabi*
12 | Learn to Ask Better Questions

03

PRACTICE THE DISCIPLINE OF "SUBOPTIMAL"

High-quality responses to errors, bad outcomes, or challenging situations move past fear or anger to focus on what comes next. Emergency providers use a three-step approach: identify and accept the issue or mistake, rapidly pivot yourself and your team to face the new reality, and learn from the event to evolve improvements for future cases. Steps one and two are performed in the moment, while step three is performed after the crisis has passed.

No matter how much thought or skill you bring to a patient's emergency care, sometimes things will still go wrong. The incorrect medication will get administered despite all existing safeguards, you'll drop a key instrument during a delicate aspect of an important procedure, or the power will go out right as multiple accident victims arrive at the ambulance bay.

The list of what can and does go wrong during a crisis is essentially endless, so preventing one hundred percent of errors, mistakes, or unlucky breaks is simply not possible.[1] When bad outcomes do occur, you need to be able to react to them in a way that moves you and your team past the initial wave of negative emotion and toward a more productive response. In this section, we consider a three-step process to recover from a setback and build stronger and more resilient systems of emergency response.

To set the stage, imagine you're called into the room of a patient who was recently placed on a ventilator for a severe asthma attack. The patient's oxygen level is dropping, and the ventilator is showing that it's getting more and more difficult to move her lungs. A quick investigation reveals that the patient had not been receiving the inhaled medications you'd ordered. Partly as a result, air is building up in her chest—an extremely dangerous situation. Without immediate action, she is at risk of suffering a ruptured lung or even cardiac arrest.

When faced with critical or rapidly changing emergent circumstances like this, typical untrained, junior-level responses are based on initial emotional surges of either fear or anger. Fear-based responses can lead to running away from the emergency—by ignoring it or denying it exists—or catastrophizing and giving up. Anger-based responses might be directed internally with self-flagellation and negative self-talk, or externally with excessive focus on something or someone outside your control whom you believe to be at fault.

Sobbing in fear or pretending nothing has happened and returning to whatever you were doing are not the right answers; neither are angrily shaking the ventilator or yelling at yourself or anyone else. You only have a set amount of time before this situation become irreversibly critical, and time spent on emotional tilt in either fear or anger is time stolen from actually responding to the crisis.

These initial, emotionally reactive responses are understandable. They occur naturally in untrained individuals as "protective" mechanisms to avoid the perceived stress of facing a crisis head on. During the course of an emergency though, they are counterproductive and potentially even dangerous. They must be trained out, and better responses must be trained in. Specifically, as you become a more experienced provider, your goal is to move past the initial emotional surge and rapidly begin to focus on what happened and how you can address it.

A skilled response to a bad outcome involves three parts: labeling, processing, and learning. The labeling and processing parts collectively form the acute phase of response immediately after the event, while learning takes place later when it is safer to dig into why things happened the way they did.

The first step in responding to a bad outcome is labeling the situation for what it is. Your goal in this step is to alert the team that your situation has changed and acknowledge the difficulty you must all now face, without giving in to distress or distraction.

Personally, when I perform the labeling part of a response, I begin by saying, "Well, this is suboptimal." Labeling something as "suboptimal" acknowledges the challenging nature of what is happening without pulling me or my team off-line the way that calling it "horrible" or "hopeless" might.

The word "suboptimal" also adds a little bit of lightheartedness and space to the situation. Standing in the emergency department covered in blood and vomit with yet another screaming patient rolling in can be a stressful situation, to put it mildly. Calling a critical failure like an unstable ventilated patient "suboptimal" is just ridiculously understated enough to help maintain the proper focus and balance between being not too tight and not too loose.

Of course, there is nothing particularly magical about the phrase "This is suboptimal," and you should experiment with different phrase to find one that suits you best. Whatever you choose, calm delivery in an even tone is crucial to convey both the urgency of the situation and your faith in your team's ability to respond.[2]

The second step in processing a challenging (read "suboptimal") situation is to identify your new priorities and pivot your team into their new roles and actions. A potentially counterintuitive first move in this process is the action of pausing and breathing. It might seem like immediate action is always necessary after a bad outcome, but often the initial thoughts that dominate after a setback are blunt and reactive concepts that lack skill or nuance.

Taking a moment to pause and breathe gives the physiologic signals of stress generated by your initial emotions time to wash out of your body. Once these fight-or-flight feelings have passed, you will likely be capable of producing more flexible and efficient ideas.

Depending on the nature of the emergency, you might not have time to safely pause and wash out the stress because an immediate response is required. In this case, you can dovetail the first part of your response (labeling the situation as suboptimal) into pre-prepared algorithms or protocols like the A-B-C approach used in critical resuscitations. These systems can serve as intelligent defaults to guide your team's initial actions when there really is no time to think.

Once you have identified the planned response—either immediate action or a more nuanced approach—your next job during the processing phase is orienting your team to their new actions. Simple, direct commands are important, as is explicitly sharing your mental model with your team to ensure everyone is on the same page. Calm delivery is again key, and closed-loop communication—in which the receiver echoes back key information—can be extremely useful.

Personally, I use a standard format statement when reorienting my team after a challenging event, a statement that explicitly identifies the new most important action. Continuing the asthma example, this would take the form of: "Team, our priority here is to disconnect the ventilator and decompress the lungs." This communication starts with the intended recipient—here, the whole team—and explicitly labels the most important next action that we need to take.

After stating the priority, you should ensure understanding via closed-loop communication with key members of the team. For example, you might say, "Amy, please disconnect the vent and press down on the chest." To close the loop, your teammate Amy would then respond, "Disconnecting vent. Pressing on chest."

Alternatively, depending on the situation, you could use this time to ask for dissenting opinions. Again, experiment to find the phrasing that feels most natural and efficient for you while remaining calm and directing your team's attention to their next most important task.

Finally, once we have cleared the acute phase of the event, the last step of this process is to analyze what happened and try to derive reusable lessons for future cases. Before the situation and your initial wave of emotions about it have cleared, diving into deep learning or making sweeping changes to protocols is extremely unlikely to yield useful results. The same can be said for trying to examine the event years later, when important details might have been lost or key participants might be unavailable.

If the crux of the situation can be easily identified, it's often sufficient to take two to five minutes after clearing the event to debrief and generate ideas for future work. Before the debrief, encourage your team members to hydrate, visit the bathroom, or otherwise take a moment to regroup. This will usually result in calmer, more mentally flexible individuals who generate better ideas than attempting an immediate debrief without taking a break. This is especially important after emotionally challenging cases when individuals may need to process their thoughts before being able to share them.

If the situation is more complex, or if addressing it requires more resources than can safely be devoted to debriefing at the moment, you can perform a post hoc analysis at a later time. Taking a moment to write down basic notes on your thought processes at the time may help you and your team better reflect on what happened and what you were thinking during and after the event.

Combining different types of post-event learning protocols can result in greater efficacy. Continuing the asthma example, you might choose to take two minutes after the patient is recovered to review protocols for sick asthmatic patients and gather basic ideas on what might have happened. After the shift, you could trigger a more formal root cause analysis to try to identify where communication about medication orders went wrong, or develop situation-based checklists or specific protocols to improve future care of asthmatic patients on ventilators.[3]

Take Action

The best way to train this three-step process of recovering from a bad outcome is to practice it during low-impact events. When something goes wrong in your day-to-day life, practice saying out loud, "Well, this is suboptimal." Then take a breath or two. Identify and say out loud what your next priority is, then move immediately to do it. After the situation has stabilized, do a quick debrief with anyone involved to see if there is anything to learn.

Experiment with different variations of the process and iterate to find what feels most natural to you when stress is low. That will help you deploy the process later in more serious situations. You don't have to apply the whole process to every event. Try parts of it alone or in combination to highlight what feels right and what still needs work.

After trying the process in low-stress situations, you can start bringing it to bear in more complicated emergencies with higher stakes. It will be important to continue iterating and experimenting during this transition, since transferring learning from low-stakes to high-stakes situations is never perfect.

See Also

04 | Apply Graduated Pressure

16 | Commit to Never Waste Suffering

22 | Find Your Locus of Control

04

APPLY GRADUATED PRESSURE

Building your emergency mind requires deliberately practicing skills in pressure-filled situations, not just in calm conditions. Excessive stress early in learning, however, is counterproductive and potentially even dangerous. Emergency providers utilize graduated-pressure protocols to first learn the basics of a skill then adapt it in increasingly pressurized environments. One of the key advantages of this approach is its ability to sequentially identify which components of a system fail at which levels of stress, and which components are ready to be deployed.

Pressure makes everything more difficult to accomplish. If you've ever tried to perform a simple task while being yelled at— even something as straight-forward as tying your shoes—it rapidly becomes clear that all tasks can become significantly more challenging when the heat is on. As time frames shorten, consequences grow, and uncertainty rises, even highly trained individuals can struggle to maintain performance and bring their top skill levels to bear on a situation.

If you need a technique to function well during a crisis, it's not enough to practice it only in a controlled environment. Testing protocols and systems under real-world pressure is a critical component of preparing to perform during emergencies. However, applying too much stress too quickly can limit learning or even lead to dangerous conditions. For example, practicing a new type of swing against a professional-level baseball pitcher could lead to bad habits or serious injuries. Practicing breath-holding techniques for freediving in even shallow water can have deadly consequences. To find that middle ground where training is effective but safe, emergency medical providers apply the concept of graduated pressure to slowly and safely test and improve a skill before relying on it during a true crisis.

Applying graduated pressure involves first seeking to understand a concept in a friendly, ultra-low-stakes environment. Then, when you understand the basics of the skill, you practice deploying it multiple times in conditions of increasing difficulty. Ultimately these conditions may mimic or even exceed the pressure of the real-life target environment in which you plan to perform.

For example, when learning to place an ultrasound-guided central line (a long intravenous catheter placed into the large subclavian, internal jugular, or femoral veins), you usually start by walking through the procedure on a plastic simulator that mimics the anatomy of a real patient.[1] Once you have a deep understanding of the basics and you are regularly succeeding at placing lines in low-stress environments, you can begin to apply more and more pressure. You might practice placing a line on a simulator in a noisy or antagonistic environment, or you might assist a more senior provider in placing a line on a live patient. Eventually, you will become the primary operator and place central lines in live patients under a variety of controlled and non-controlled environments.

While it's tempting to chart progress through graduated-pressure iterations by identifying the scenarios in which you succeed, the true magic of practice with graduated pressure comes from the way you encounter failures and setbacks during the repetitions.[2] If you put a system under extreme stress from the beginning—like attempting to hit a fastball from the first at-bat—the system will break at multiple points without providing useful information on exactly what went wrong. You know you struck out, but you have no idea why or what to do to improve your next time at bat.

Instead, when you gradually increase the pressure in your learning environment, each iteration offers the opportunity to find a previously unseen weakness in your understanding or execution of the technique and the opportunity to address it. In this way, as you slowly increase the speed of the pitches, you can work sequentially on reading the pitch, improving the arc of your swing, maximizing the biomechanics of your stance, etc.

Back in the ER, imagine you need to place a central line into a crashing trauma patient. Without proper training, the probable resulting failure would be just as likely to result from not knowing where the equipment was stored as from a fundamental flaw in your understanding of how to modify a crucial part of the procedure. Figuring out exactly why the procedure failed and what to do about it would be nearly impossible, since your operator-procedure dyad would have failed in so many locations.

Conversely, if you had trained using graduated pressure, you would have taken care of the simple things—like where the central-line kit was stored—during dry-run practice. Eliminating minor stumbling blocks like this early on leaves more mental energy available to actually place the line and improves your chances of success. Hopefully, you would place it correctly. But even if not, you would be better poised to learn what went wrong and process the event for use in subsequent attempts.

As author James Clear writes, "The Goldilocks Rule states that humans experience peak motivation when working on tasks that are right on the edge of their current abilities. Not too hard. Not too easy. Just right."[3] Finding the edge where your skills are at their limits and your performance is raw and imperfect over and over allows you to iterate, experiment, and progressively improve your techniques. In this way, you can learn from all your struggles as opposed to being crushed by them.

Take Action

One of the best ways you can execute graduated-pressure training is through visualization practice, which is the active mental rehearsal of a process in order to improve subsequent real-world performance. Mental visualization practice is always accessible, and you can alter the pressure you bring to bear in infinite ways.

To start, close your eyes and visualize the step-by-step execution of a particular skill, such as the insertion of a central line. Don't just visualize the critical points like inserting the needle, visualize every step from starting with opening the kit to finishing by placing the final dressing. Then, when you are ready to practice with graduated pressure, add distracting or difficult elements to your visualization by mentally walking through the procedure while also visualizing a screaming family member, multiple alarms going off, or other high-pressure elements.

If your visualization crumbles, you can note where and why it failed, and study or practice to train that particular element. If it succeeds, you can celebrate, then try again with even more mental pressure added to the mix.

Personally, a technique I use is to "borrow" pressure from other events. A key component of how you feel pressure is the activity of your sympathetic nervous system, which readies your body for stress by performing tasks like increasing your heart rate, speeding up your breathing, and making you sweat. To facilitate pressure training, you can take advantage of other situations that generate similar physiologic responses and mentally rehearse techniques when your sympathetic system is already revved up.

For example, you could pause and visualize placing a central line at the end of a hard workout. Initially you could practice visualizing a process after mild exertion. Then, the harder your physical exertion, the more revved up your physiology would be and the higher the pressure you would be simulating. With practice, borrowing pressure like this will increase the number of repetitions you're able to execute in pressurized situations before an actual crisis occurs.

See Also
06 | Practice *Wabi-Sabi*
08 | Become Comfortable with Uncertainty
16 | Commit to Never Waste Suffering

05

TRAIN YOUR TIRED MOVES

Your "tired moves" are the techniques and protocols that function not only when you're at full capacity, but when you or your team are exhausted. Overtraining these basic techniques produces a core structure that is resilient to stress and lays a foundation upon which more advanced practices can be based. Identifying which techniques are tired moves should involve leveraging both your personal experience and the aggregate analysis of others to determine what methods yield high success rates under extreme pressure.

Ten hours into your shift, the emergency radio goes off with a call from an ambulance crew about to arrive. They are carrying an unresponsive child who was struck by a car while riding her bike. It has been a challenging shift, and as you move into the resuscitation bay, you take stock of the situation: you're feeling rough, your coffee is long gone, and your scrubs are bloodied.

You and your team have been under significant cognitive and physical loads for many hours. The fatigue is palpable, but emergencies happen on their own schedule, not on yours. Certainly, optimizing ratios of rest and performance, improving nutrition and hydration, and balancing stress and recovery are important and worthwhile goals. But if you want to be able to perform under pressure, you need to learn to play tired.

In moments like this, when you and your team must press on despite depleted reserves, you will rely not on your flashiest or most sophisticated tools, but on your "tired moves:" the skills, protocols, and techniques you have overtrained to the point that you could do them in your sleep. Put succinctly, your tired moves continue to work even when you are exhausted.

The first time I heard the concept of "tired moves" called explicitly by that name was in a jiu-jitsu class. I had just finished a long match in which I had attempted and failed to escape a bad position using a sophisticated technique I clearly had not fully understood.

Seeing me flounder, one of the coaches called me over and explained the concept to me something like this: "Look. Some things are great moves, but you can only pull them off in the beginning of your match when you're 100 percent fresh. You have to think about what you can actually do when you're dead tired, later in the round. These are your tired moves—and you have to drill those moves, not just the flashy ones."[1]

In the emergency department, an important tired move is successfully delivering breaths to a patient using a bag-valve mask (BVM) system. Using a BVM to assist a patient's breathing—called "bagging" the patient—is a basic skill, typically one of the first taught in airway management sessions. It certainly does not have the sophistication of more advanced techniques like placing a breathing tube using a flexible fiber-optic camera, but it functions even when the electricity has failed, or when the more advanced equipment is broken.[2]

Whether your goal is ventilating a patient or escaping to a better position in jiu-jitsu, how do you determine what skills should be trained and overtrained as tired moves? The two key methods are personal practice and aggregate analysis. Individuals and teams devoted to improving their performance under pressure should develop ways to utilize each of these methods, and preferably both together.

First, personal practice involves attempting to perform different skills in high-pressure and high-fatigue situations and seeing for yourself what works and what does not. Emergency departments might employ simulation labs to create near-real-life situations, while martial artists might use sparring or training matches. Alternating between training a skill in low-stress, calm environments when you're fresh and in higher-stress environments when you're tired can be especially helpful. Incorporating elements of stress and fatigue can be accomplished through a variety of means including training skills immediately after strenuous physical exercise or running simulations both at the beginning and the end of long periods of exertion to compare responses.

If you don't have immediate access to an external testing ground—or if real-life testing is too dangerous—you can run mental simulations in which you visualize performing a technique under varying scenarios and attempt to identify where further training is needed. Postmortem visualization, in which you start with the assumption that you have failed at a task and then work backward to visualize why, can be particularly useful in identifying tired moves.[3]

Second, aggregate analysis involves developing arsenals of tired moves by mining the experiences of groups that have deployed different techniques in a variety of real-life situations. As part of an after-action debrief, you can ask which protocols and techniques kept functioning (or even improved) when exhaustion set in, and which ones broke down or failed.

Armed with the knowledge of what actually holds up under pressure, you can decide either to overtrain these actions, or design experiments for new ideas that might fill existing holes. Of course, developing tired moves through aggregate analysis only works if you have access to data on what functions well and what does not. Teams and institutions should therefore devote resources to capturing data on which techniques worked best in high-fatigue environments.

Regardless of the method you use, to function during an emergency you need to proactively train your tired moves now, while you're fresh. Training basic skills under pressure might not be the most fun or exciting aspect of improving your performance during a crisis, but when you are truly deep in the dirt and struggling under the weight of an emergency, you will be happy you did it.

Take Action

Start by defining the scenario for which you will be training tired moves. Perhaps you are an emergency provider training to place a breathing tube to control a patient's airway, or a helicopter pilot attempting to land in heavy fog. The more information you have on the environment in which you're likely to practice and the levels of strain you're likely to encounter, the better prepared your tired moves will be. If you don't have or cannot obtain accurate information on the expected environment, you should overestimate the levels of stress for this exercise.

Once you've identified your goals, reflect on any previous personal experience you might have in the exact situation or in similar ones. What challenges did you face with your standard operating procedures, and what backup moves might have worked? Are there any obvious techniques that either fail wildly or show significant promise? To harness this type of information moving forward, you might set up recording mechanisms to keep track of what works well and what crumbles under pressure and fatigue. One way to do this is to designate a provider not otherwise involved in a case to observe you functioning under high-fatigue conditions and provide external feedback on how your tired moves held up.

Whether or not you have personal experience, you will also want to analyze records of other operators performing in similar circumstances. Where formal databases or mission logs exist, these should be studied in depth.[4] Where data is scarce, the experiences of individual operators could be studied, though this involves potential biases related to small sample sizes and difficulties with accurate recall. In this case, it can be particularly useful to ask a more seasoned operator what basic skills they do differently now than at the beginning of their careers, and why they changed how they perform them.

See Also

17 | Humans Not Robots

19 | Favor Praxis Over Theory

20 | Rapidly Accept Reality

II

HANDLING UNCERTAINTY AND IMPERFECTION

06

PRACTICE *WABI-SABI*

Wabi-sabi embodies the concept that natural things are inherently imperfect, impermanent, and incomplete. Working with the wabi-sabi nature of the universe during an emergency helps you move past an unproductive and illogical need for perfect answers or permanent, unchanging solutions in order to focus on what actually works. Plans and teams built with wabi-sabi in mind are flexible and adaptive, resilient to failures of individual components, and more likely to succeed under pressure.

The Japanese concept of *wabi-sabi* explores the ideas that nothing is permanent, nothing is perfect, and nothing is complete. Traditionally applied to the realm of art and design, *wabi-sabi* evokes the dynamic natural world and the inherent cycle of growth, change, and decay. Its "opposite" would be a static and artificial situation, unchanging rules, and rigid structures.[1]

When you need to perform during a crisis, a *wabi-sabi* mindset will help you focus on growth and improvement, accept uncertainty, and fluidly adapt to changing circumstances. By comparison, ignoring the *wabi-sabi* nature of life results in an inflexible approach that makes you more likely to underperform or even collapse when the pressure is on.

Consider for example an elderly man who presents for emergency care because he has trouble walking and an elevated blood pressure. If you hold a "fixed" or non-*wabi-sabi* view of the world, you might focus on the "textbook answer" of 120/80 mmHg as an optimal blood pressure and be tempted to immediately decrease his blood pressure toward that goal. Taking a *wabi-sabi* worldview, you would note that there is no absolute "perfect" blood pressure, and that this patient's optimal blood pressure depends upon on his specific situation.

If his trouble walking is caused by dizziness from high blood pressure (perhaps via a hypertensive encephalopathy), then decreasing the blood pressure slowly by around twenty percent would typically be a good treatment. However, if his difficulty walking is caused by an acute ischemic stroke, then the elevated blood pressure might be his body's attempt to maintain a high enough perfusion pressure to "push" blood past the blockage. Allowing the blood pressure to autoregulate and remain high could be a better solution in this case. Regardless of the underlying cause, considering both the abstract "ideal" blood pressure and the details of this particular situation will likely result in a better outcome than rigidly adhering to any one standard playbook in a vacuum.

To further explore how *wabi-sabi* can help you and your team perform better under pressure, let's consider each of its main aspects—impermanence, imperfection, and incompleteness.[2]

First, impermanence. Nothing in life, not even you nor I, is permanent. If you recognize and accept this impermanence, you can build flexible plans that adapt to changing needs and are resilient to stressors. Conversely, if you deny that situations change, you create a potentially dangerous schism between your view of the universe and the actual reality around you. As this gap increases, the solutions and plans you had generated before reality changed will rapidly be made ineffective, if not counterproductive or dangerous. For example, if you were flying a plane and an engine fails, you wouldn't waste time holding onto a mental model of a plane with multiple working engines. Instead, you would want to adjust to the new reality as rapidly as possible and develop a way to fly the plane with whatever engines you have left.

In the emergency department, the emergence of a new disease, such as COVID-19, requires protocols and systems of care that can rapidly evolve to keep pace with new information and changing practices. Even in a "steady state" of emergency care outside an acute pandemic, new techniques and new ideas need to be continually absorbed and integrated into your existing protocols. If your view of how to practice medicine is too rigid—too invested in permanence—this type of evolution will be difficult to accomplish.

Second, imperfection. Embracing the idea that nothing is perfect during a crisis helps you maintain focus on growth, rather than comparing your response to some theoretical optimum. No matter where you are in your training, you doubtlessly want to perform at your best during an emergency. However, when less than-perfect events occur—and they will—it can be easy to get bogged down in what happened rather than stay focused on what to do next. As a result, you risk further mistakes by fixating on imperfections or missed opportunities.

Wabi-sabi thinking teaches you that since nothing is perfect, perfection cannot and should not be your goal during a crisis. Instead, you can focus on performing at your absolute best and continuing to grow with each event you encounter. This might mean accepting a "good enough" solution you can actually accomplish, as opposed to being paralyzed while you look for the "perfect" solution.[3] After a crisis is complete, you evaluate yourself not only against set standards but also against your own prior attempts. In this way you'll recognize how far you've come while staying focused on what needs to improve next.

Finally, incompletion. You need to recognize that individuals and systems never stop growing and changing; nothing is ever complete. You will never have the complete answer on how to perform, since there is no total final answer. Growth, iteration, and experimentation should therefore be the norm for your teams, and you should welcome rather than resist changes in how you operate. You should always be willing to learn new ways to perform during a crisis, to update your mental models, and to seek feedback on how to do better. This applies both to beginners and more skilled practitioners alike; even the most masterful musician continues to tune her instrument before every performance.

Holding this in mind helps you work to eliminate any trace of the "sacred way that things are done here" mentality, which can limit creative thinking and breed stagnation. Accepting that nothing is ever complete, you should work to develop a culture that consistently encourages new and better ways to respond to emergencies. Removing obsolete mental models in favor of more effective ones should be rewarded, even if those obsolete mental models were ones *you* created in the first place.

Taking these three ideas together, practicing *wabi-sabi* means becoming a dedicated and lifelong student of your craft. You do not look for perfection, for completeness of knowledge, or for solutions that are "forever" answers. Instead, as you build your emergency mind, you focus on improving your performance and doing the best you can with what you have. You accept uncertainty and change, since they are omnipresent, and you devote yourself to growing with every crisis you encounter.

Take Action

A good way to begin training a *wabi-sabi* mindset is to take a critical look into the protocols and patterns you currently use. Identify which systems around you are based on artificial ideas of perfection, permanence, or completeness, and which are based in the principles of *wabi-sabi*. How well do these different types of systems function when placed under pressure?

If you discover than an entire system hinges on one factor going "perfectly," imagine what would happen if that single factor breaks down. How would you recover and move on? Are there contingency plans or alternative approaches you should put in place now? For example, if a key piece of software your company uses runs entirely on one server, what happens when that server goes down? If the door to a room containing critical backup equipment is "always" unlocked, what happens when it accidentally gets locked? Proactively thinking through these questions now, before an emergency happens, will yield dividends when you are called on to act under pressure.

In general, when you plan an approach to a problem, hope for the best but design with the assumption that some things will fail or be imperfect. Train yourself to build these ideas in from the beginning, and proactively spend time with your backup plans. When circumstances do force you onto a different path, sometimes actually saying *"wabi-sabi"* out loud can help you let go of your need for permanence and better allow you to actively update your view of the world.

See Also

08 | Become Comfortable with Uncertainty
10 | Make "Plan B" Part of the Plan
20 | Rapidly Accept Reality

07

UNDERSTAND FALLIBILITY AND COGNITIVE BIAS

Cognitive biases reflect assumptions your brain makes below the level of conscious thought in order to simplify processing of the often-complex reality around you. These assumptions frequently have unintended consequences and can lead to systematic errors in thought and performance during a crisis. Exploring how cognitive biases subtly or overtly alter your seemingly logical efforts at making decisions is the first step in accounting for their effects. Every cognitive bias you are able to recognize is one you can attempt to adjust for while making decisions under pressure.

As a human being, your brain is capable of deep and sophisticated analyses across a variety of environments both in and out of emergency situations. Your brain also is inherently imperfect and prone to multiple types of errors, especially when placed under pressure. Among these imperfections are cognitive biases—systematic deviations from perfectly rational decision making that reproducibly lead to analytic errors with potentially disastrous results.

Cognitive biases are assumptions about the reality around you that your brain makes below the level of your conscious control. These assumptions seem to exist to lighten the computational load of rapid and complex decision making. When the proverbial saber-toothed tiger is bearing down on you, cognitive biases can help simplify choices and speed up reaction times. However, if left unchecked, these unconscious shortcuts can have wide ranging and potentially severe consequences in how individuals and teams perform during a crisis.

Understanding the basics of how cognitive biases function is crucial to mitigating their effects and improving your performance during an emergency.[1] While fully exploring the variety of cognitive biases that have been identified is beyond the scope of this book, every cognitive bias you recognize and explore can help you improve how you and your team function. In this section we will review three cognitive biases commonly encountered when performing under pressure: anchoring bias, confirmation bias, and recency bias.

Anchoring bias describes the cognitive error you make when you tend to give more weight to information arriving early in a situation compared to information arriving later—regardless of the relative quality or relevance of that initial information. Whatever data is presented to you first when you start to look at a situation can form an "anchor" and it becomes significantly more challenging to alter your mental course away from this anchor than it logically should be.

A classic example of anchoring bias in emergency medicine is "triage bias," where whatever the first impression you develop, or are given, about a patient tends to influence all subsequent providers seeing that patient. For example, imagine two patients presenting for emergency care with aching jaw pain that occasionally extends down to their chest. Differences in how the intake providers label the chart—"jaw pain" vs. "chest pain," for example—create anchors that might result in significant differences in how the patients are treated.

Despite telling very similar stories, one patient might be routed to a minor injury area for jaw pain, while the other is brought more rapidly to an area better capable of cardiac workups. Even if the patients are brought to the same location, as the next provider to see them, you might treat them different based on the initial complaint of jaw vs. chest pain.

Confirmation bias is closely related to anchoring bias. It describes the cognitive error you make when you're more likely to believe information that supports your current hypothesis or course of action and conversely more likely to discount information that suggests you might be incorrect. While logically you should weigh each new piece of information during a crisis on its own merits, confirmation bias suggests that you often subtly (or greatly) prefer coherence with your existing theory over absolute truth.

A significant and unfortunate instance of confirmation bias can come into play when you are physically lost. Imagine a group hiking in the mountains that unknowingly had drifted off the intended path. If the individuals in the groups still believe themselves to be heading in the right direction, they will often ignore signs that they may be lost and may bend the information they're gathering to "confirm" their current course.

In the emergency department, your equivalent to a "hiking path" is the mental trail of what you think your patient is experiencing and what you're planning to do about it. Getting lost is akin to misdiagnosing the problem. When you're convinced you understand what's happening to your patient, confirmation bias says you will tend to ignore signs pointing to alternate potential diagnoses and favor information that supports your current hypothesis.

In essence, confirmation bias is about preferring to maintain one's current mental model (that you are on the right path) over a new mental model (that you are lost or mistaken), even when there is no outside logical reason to do so. Uninterested observers who do not "own" a particular mental model do not feel a cost to changing their mind. Consequently, they are less likely to make confirmation errors compared to the person whose beliefs are being confirmed or disproven.

Finally, recency bias describes the cognitive error you make when you give more weight to things that have happened recently simply because they are more easily available for mental recall. Since whatever happened recently might not be a good predictor of what is about to happen, recency bias can significantly skew emergency responses based on small sample sizes or personal experience. The equally important flip side of recency bias is subconsciously discounting things you have never personally seen or experienced, believing they are less likely to occur than they actually are.

During one of my first years after residency training, I provided emergency care to a patient who presented with a sore throat. Initially, there was nothing special about the case—plenty of people come to emergency centers with throat pain, and the vast majority are generally healthy and leave after minor treatment. This patient though, was suffering from acute epiglottitis—a rare and exceedingly dangerous type of airway infection that can rapidly progress and stop the patient from breathing.

Intellectually, I knew what epiglottitis was, but in part because I had no personal experience with it, my team and I struggled to arrive at the correct diagnosis. Recency bias nudged me toward favoring other diagnoses I had seen, such as like strep throat or viral pharyngitis. As the infection in this patient's throat progressed rapidly, he had a very complicated course and ultimately suffered a respiratory arrest. Thankfully, we eventually were able to secure his airway, and he made a full recovery.

For the several months after treating that patient, every time I saw a someone presenting with a sore throat, I found myself briefly convinced they were suffering from epiglottitis. While the baseline prevalence of epiglottitis had not altered, the share of my "brain space" it occupied had changed drastically due in large part to the effects of recency bias. It required my conscious effort and recognition of the recency bias effect for me to return to a more useful and accurate balance that reflected the true prevalence of what is likely (non-threatening viral infections) and what is rare and potentially dangerous (epiglottitis).

Take Action

The first time I learned about cognitive biases, I remember thinking how interesting it was that everyone else's minds worked that way; not my mind, of course, just everyone else's. The truth, though, is that each one of us is affected by cognitive biases—none of our minds are perfectly rational. This means that everyone is fallible, including me and including you. Knowing that, what can you do about it? While psychology experts suggest that it probably isn't possible to fully eliminate cognitive biases, there are things that you can do to address them.

First, simply knowing that cognitive biases exist can help you hold a view of reality that includes having a limited, sometimes irrational brain. This can make it easier for you to learn about a part of your mind that is not easily accessible, and also improve the likelihood that you will accept help from others, even if you feel you might not need it. For example, if a teammate challenges your logic or points out a potential flaw in your reasoning, being aware of cognitive biases can make you more likely to consider your team-mate's point of view.

Second, knowing about individual cognitive biases can allow you to generate strategies to address and potentially overcome them. In the case of anchoring bias, an easy strategy is to slightly alter the chief complaint on a patient's chart and notice if that change alters your mental model of the patient. In the case of confirmation bias, an important strategy is to actively seek disconfirming evidence, especially when the decision has high levels of potential impact. For example, prior to stating that efforts should be terminated in a cardiac arrest, it is common for the leader of the resuscitation team to ask for help identifying potential blind spots. Personally, I ask, "Team, what am I *not* seeing?" In this way, the team will focus on disconfirming the hypothesis (and finding another way to restart the patient's heart) rather than agreeing automatically that there is no more to be done.

In the case of recency bias, teams can work to pay extra attention to typical rates of events from large sample sizes as opposed to their own limited experience.[2] Alternatively, the "What are we not seeing?" question could also be used to help identify where recency bias was discounting a potential explanation of the crisis.

Finally, running a particularly critical decision through an external decision-support structure—such as a checklist or a group of fellow experts—is crucial to help mitigate cognitive biases.[3]

One of the most important decision-support tools we use in the emergency department is the "time out," a structured pause immediately before the start of a crucial procedure. During the time out, all individuals who will be involved in the procedure gather together in the place where the procedure will be performed. They discuss the details of the planned procedure, confirm that the intended procedure matches the proposed underlying purpose, and discuss any expected deviations that might occur.

Doing this "group mental walk-through" not only ensures that you are performing the right procedure on the right patient at the right time, but also gives you another opportunity to check your logic and reasoning and hunt for any remaining bias.

See Also

09 | Harness the Wisdom of the Room

13 | Eliminate Unnecessary Opportunities for Failure

17 | Humans Not Robots

08

BECOME COMFORTABLE WITH UNCERTAINTY

Every emergency involves uncertainty, so learning to operate under uncertain conditions is crucial to an effective emergency response. While some types of uncertainty are obvious, other types are more subtle and require active awareness to identify. Your goal is not the elimination of uncertainty, but efficient functioning given uncertain conditions. Understanding this distinction will help you prioritize and fine tune your actions under varying degrees of uncertainty.

Learning to operate successfully under conditions of uncertainty is fundamental to building your emergency mind; requiring certainty before action often leads to unacceptable or even fatal delays. Consider for example a young woman coming into your emergency department gasping for air and covered in an itchy rash after eating something she thinks might have contained shellfish, to which she is allergic. Most likely, she is having a severe allergic reaction, so you need to act immediately to stabilize her before her reaction progresses to shock or airway compromise. You don't have time to call the local restaurant where she just ate to confirm that the soup does, in fact, have shrimp in it. If you required complete certainty before you acted in this case, your patient might suffer or die.

Not all situations you face will have such stark distinctions between seeking more clarity and acting, but all emergencies *will* involve some degree of uncertainty. To operate successfully during a crisis, you must become comfortable acting with limited or imperfect information. As firefighter and author Peter Leschak put it, "You must not merely tolerate uncertainty, you must savor it. Or you won't last long."[1]

A first step toward increasing your comfort with uncertainty is to explore the explicit and implicit ways in which uncertainty can come into play during a crisis. Explicit uncertainty describes an obvious knowledge gap, while implicit uncertainty is less obvious and requires conscious work to identify and address.

Explicit uncertainty occurs when you know you lack understanding or are missing a particular piece of information. This uncertainty might involve details of the issue you're facing, your available response options, the likely outcomes of particular actions, or combinations of all three.

Imagine for example that you are sailing a small boat with family and friends when you receive an emergency radio communication about an incoming rouge wave. In this situation, explicit uncertainty abounds: Where exactly is the wave heading? Is it coming toward you? If so, how long do you have, and which types of evasive actions could you possibly employ? Of those potential options, which direction should you choose to sail? Uncertainty here is explicit.

By comparison, implicit uncertainty can be substantially more hidden and you may have to purposefully look for it. One important example of implicit or hidden uncertainty is the concept of test error. When you perform a medical test, you tend to take the results as fact and truly representative of reality. However, since no test is perfect, the result you get is a bit more like a guess of what actually is happening. Depending on the situation, that guess might be a good guess or a bad guess, but either way it's a guess, not the absolute truth.

Underestimating the uncertainty that comes with test results can lead to significant diagnostic and treatment errors. This can be tricky to understand, so let's make it more concrete. Consider what happens when you run a test to measure the sodium level in a patient's blood. In the emergency department, we run this test routinely as part of every basic metabolic panel along with tests of kidney function, blood glucose, etc.

Sodium measurements are generally fairly accurate, and the "true" value of the patient's sodium is typically thought to be within 1-2 mEq/L of the reported value in most cases.[2] While this level of uncertainty is generally small enough to be irrelevant, if your entire treatment plan depends on accurately measuring your patient's sodium level, then the uncertainty might make a significant difference in how you choose to act.

Aside from the uncertainty when a test is "behaving normally," tests can also sometimes be "tricked" by other factors. In the case of measuring sodium, elevated levels of blood glucose distort test results markedly, leading to falsely low sodium readings. Without awareness of the hidden uncertainty in these test results, treatment plans might be ineffective or even potentially harmful.[3]

Since handling both explicit and implicit uncertainty are such important parts of performing during a crisis, how can you learn to "savor the uncertainty" as Leschak suggests? First, recognize that getting rid of uncertainty is not always the goal; responding to the emergency is. You don't always need to remove uncertainty to address the emergency. You just need to learn to be comfortable with the uncertainty you face.

For example, suppose you're working in an emergency department and receive a paramedic call-in for an adult male who seems to have suffered a drug overdose. The paramedics are not sure of the man's age or name, but he was found nearly unconscious next to some drug paraphernalia and he is not breathing well. In this case, identifying the patient's name or age is not actually relevant—eliminating this uncertainty does not change what you need to do to take care of him. What is important is supporting the patient's breathing and treating potential causes of his altered mental status. Similarly, returning to the example of the boat, no matter what course the wave is taking, you should put on your life jacket.

Second, you can work to learn the physiological signs of uncertainty in your own body and mind. When faced with decisions in uncertain conditions, do you tense up? Do you tend to experience abdominal pain? Are you short with friends or coworkers? Sometimes what really is uncomfortable is not the uncertainty itself, but how you have conditioned your body to react to it.

Addressing your body's response can often help mitigate the fear of uncertainty. This, in turn, can help you generate a more rational response to the uncertain conditions. To accomplish this, some providers use deep breathing techniques to counter uncertainty-induced shortness of breath. Others mentally walk through their bodies and visualize "unlocking" tight muscles. Personally, I take my own pulse at my right wrist, which helps me process my elevated heart rate as a sign of readiness, not of fear.

Whatever technique you use, how you interpret these physiological signals is a choice. After all, the mystery of not knowing what's around the next curve is mentally mapped to fear by some and to adventure by others. Learning to re-interpret bodily sensations in a more favorable light is a skill you can train.[4]

Finally, where possible, you can identify potential outcomes and train for contingencies. If you have developed well-tested backup plans with which you feel confident and prepared, then you are functionally more tolerant of uncertainty. Becoming excellent at airway control and ventilator management for example, allows you to better tolerate the uncertainty of how to help an individual who is short of breath. You know that if the situation deteriorates further, you will be in a good position to provide care.

Becoming comfortable with uncertainty is not something you can learn from someone else, the way a more senior provider can teach you pharmacology or the steps of a particular procedure. Instead, learning to enjoy performing under uncertain conditions is a skill you must take responsibility for and consciously study and train. As mindfulness expert Jon Kabat-Zinn famously said, "You can't stop the waves, but you can learn to surf."

Take Action

Your goal in handling uncertainty is not to eliminate it, but to function well in its presence. An important first step is to examine what you do currently. Identify the situations in which you typically try to eliminate uncertainty and those times in which you're comfortable acting in its presence. Then work to identify the signs and symptoms of how you currently process uncertainty. When you find yourself in situations with high degrees of uncertainty, make notes about what you feel physically and mentally. Practice holding steady in the face of these experiences and ask yourself if your actions are designed to actually achieve your goals or simply to eliminate unpleasant feelings.

Once you have a solid grasp on how you currently experience and respond to uncertainty, you can start to expand your comfort in its presence. Experiment with different techniques in low-stakes situations, like using deep breathing to counter the physical feelings uncertainty may bring when you're opening an email containing a medical test result. Finally, in situations where you know you will face uncertainty—like a patient with a cardiac arrest for example—train and overtrain your basic skills to improve your response times.

See Also
04 | Apply Graduated Pressure
06 | Practice *Wabi-Sabi*
14 | Decide to Not Decide

09

HARNESS THE WISDOM OF THE ROOM

As an individual, your understanding of what's happening during an emergency is inherently limited to what you personally can observe and what data you are directly exposed to. Harnessing the wisdom of the room involves building a composite model that incorporates the understanding of every individual present. This yields a more complete and more powerful vision of the crisis than your limited personal view. Galvanizing a team to work on the same problem and empowering team members to share their visions are important leadership skills for teams performing under pressure.

There's an old story that describes a group of blind individuals trying to understand what an elephant is by extrapolating the whole animal from whatever small part they are each able to personally touch and experience. One feels only the trunk and says it is flexible like a snake. Another feels only the tusk and says it is hard and sharp like a spear. Yet another feels a leg and says it must be solid and tall like a tree. Each individual only processes the small portion of the elephant in front of them. Without having combined their small pieces into a more complete mental model of what is happening, the group fails to understand they are all working with an elephant.

Like these people trying to figure out an elephant, during a crisis, you as an individual possess an incomplete and imperfect model of what is actually going on. If, however, you could combine the information and knowledge from every individual involved, the resulting composite mental model would be much more accurate and better able to represent the reality of the emergency. In other words, the wisdom of the room—defined as the ensemble of individual views of all members of the team—is better than the mental model of any one individual. In addition, the understanding you can synthesize from the wisdom of the room is often much greater than the sum of its parts.

Harnessing the wisdom of the room is useful for any decision, but during emergency situations it becomes critically important. The combination of uncertainty, impact, and pressure typically results in significant differences between a given individual's understanding and the actual reality of the situation. Revisiting our elephant metaphor, when the elephant is charging, it becomes even more important for a team to understand what they are dealing with and which way it's heading.

Decision-making expert and former professional poker player Annie Duke describes it this way, "On our own, we have just one viewpoint. That's our limitation as humans. But if we take a bunch of people with that limitation and put them together in a group, we get exposed to diverse opinions, can test alternative hypotheses, and move toward accuracy."[1]

To drive this point home during my training, I was often instructed to imagine a fictitious scenario in which the result of a critical resuscitation—whether a particular patient lived or died—depended entirely on the score you would receive on a written exam taken at the moment the patient arrived at the emergency department.[2] If everyone on your team took the exam individually, some patients would live and some would probably die as scores would vary among the test takers. However, if you were able to give the entire team one test to take together, chances are high that you could find a way to combine the available knowledge inherent in your team to score higher than any individual could alone. As a result, you would be able to deliver better care and save more patients.

So, during an active crisis, how can you best bring everyone involved together to take the same test? How can you harness the wisdom of the room and deliver it where and when it is needed? Let's dig into what leaders and team members can each do.

First, as a team leader, your goal is to actively create a culture in which everyone in the room is clear on what test you're taking and then to help everyone to take the test together. You must encourage and actively look for input from all team members, especially in teams with either implicit or explicit hierarchical structures. In cases where strong hierarchies exist, simply asking for input from the group might not be enough to elicit the information you need, as some individuals might not feel empowered to speak up, particularly if their point of view contradicts the current direction of the group.[3]

As a leader, you will frequently feel tension between your needs to process multiple points of view and to move forward rapidly with a plan. At some points during a crisis, your emphasis should be on action and the execution of your plan. At others, your emphasis might be on unifying your team's vision through open discussion. To navigate this tension, skilled leaders let their teams know verbally when only life-threatening information should be shared and conversely, when free-form ideas and suggestions of all types are welcome.[4]

As a non-leader member of a team, you can start by observing different styles of communication used by senior team members during a crisis. What protocols bring team members together to address the same test, and which shut down diverse or dissenting opinions? Any time the leader discusses their mental model of what's happening, you can contrast it with your own to identify where your training might need to be improved, or where and why you might have arrived at a different conclusion.

When you do have alternative ideas, you can and should bring them up when asked directly. Some instances might be safer than others for the team to discuss contrasting ideas broadly. As a junior team member, consider running your ideas by more seasoned teammates, or observing how and when they bring up their own opinions.

Regardless of your role on a team, being aware that your mental model likely represents only one part of the elephant is an important step toward reaching beyond your limitations to improve performance. Whenever possible, harnessing the wisdom of the room should be a top and continuing priority. The more you can galvanize your team to take the same test, the more successful you will be, no matter what crisis you face. As American author and educator Helen Keller famously said, "Alone we can do so little; together we can do so much."

Take Action

Recognizing that you have an imperfect view of the universe is a somewhat radical act. Most of us tend to believe that what we see and understand is a faithful representation of reality, and that mistakes tend to be made by someone else. Recognizing this imperfection during a crisis can give you access to lifesaving information that you might otherwise miss.

A first step in learning to harness the wisdom of the room is to ask yourself this question: "What might someone else see that I don't?" You can start asking this question informally to yourself during your day-to-day activities before deploying it under pressure. If someone arrives at a different conclusion or behaves differently than you expect, you can ask yourself what mental model they might be using to arrive at their conclusion.

A powerful question that can help you get past any initial reticence to consider an alternate viewpoint is: "What must this other person believe in order for that conclusion or action to be logical?" You can follow up by asking yourself what assumptions they might have made. What evidence did they gather and why did they interpret factors differently than I did? Which alternative conclusions did they focus on and decide to follow? Questions like these can help you widen your perspective.

Once you have some practice in processing multiple points of view, you can consider how to harness the wisdom of the room during a crisis. As stated above, differing points of view during an emergency can at times be difficult for junior members to offer or difficult for leaders to accept and process. To address this, Duke suggests that leaders could ask for information from junior team members first or ask participants to write down information which is then shared anonymously with the group.[3] In this way, individuals are more likely to express their true opinions without fear of recrimination.

Alternatively, you could explicitly ask for only dissenting information, or information that directly contradicts the main hypothesis the group currently holds. Personally, during a critical resuscitation I will often ask my team some version of, "Okay, folks.

This patient needs our collective help. What are we missing? What have we not tried yet?"

See Also

10

MAKE "PLAN B" PART OF THE PLAN

Operating during a crisis involves proactively preparing and training backup plans, since nothing goes according to your initial plan 100 percent of the time. Reframing the transition from Plan A to Plan B not as a failure but as an alternative pathway to success is a crucial part of improving individual and systems-level performance. With training and intelligent protocol design, you can create resilient operators and systems that move past stumbling blocks to find alternate ways to achieve your mission.

Your patient's oxygen saturation is dropping rapidly as you struggle to place a breathing tube. A few minutes prior, she was rushed into your ER with facial swelling and trouble breathing. She has a severe allergy to nuts and accidentally received the wrong lunch order. Unfortunately, you are having trouble placing the tube and your initial approach is just not working. Unless you pivot rapidly to a backup plan, you might lose her.

Thankfully, you had prepared for this possibility. Before implementing your initial plan, you had thought through and identified what equipment you would use in case your first pass faltered. Incorporating the information you gained from your initial attempt at securing her airway, you adjust your predetermined backup plan and move forward.

Changing to a differently shaped intubating blade, you alter the angle of your approach and call out for extra pressure on her neck. With these new maneuvers, your view of her airway improves considerably, and you successfully place the breathing tube. Watching her oxygen numbers return to normal, you gather your team to debrief to discuss what you've all learned.

Even under the best circumstances, no process or system works perfectly 100 percent of the time. Everything, including you and me, has a failure rate. During a crisis—when individuals and systems carry higher-than-normal workloads and are subject to unexpected or irregular spikes in demand—that failure rate will almost certainly increase.

When you design protocols or systems that can only be successful if their subprocesses never fail, you create structures that are inherently fragile. Conversely, preparing backup plans from the beginning—designing Plan B as part of the initial plan—generates robust systems that are much more likely to succeed during times of crisis. Preparing and being able to execute your Plan B when your initial attempt does not work is therefore an absolute necessity.

In other words, we need to view the move from Plan A to Plan B not as a failure, but as an opportunity to succeed using an alternate approach. As emergency physician Derek Monette, MD put it, "Plan B is [just] part of the plan."[1] Changing the way you view a Plan B approach like this—from failure to skillful transition—can help mitigate unnecessary self-criticism and improve focus on actually executing the plan.

When you look at Plan B as an alternative path to success, it quickly becomes obvious that you need to spend time training Plan B nearly as much, if not more, than Plan A. Immediately prior to diving into an emergency situation (such as placing a breathing tube) is certainly a good time to identify what your primary backup approach will be. However, for that backup to be an effective option, you need to have practiced it well in advance of the actual crisis.

At a systems level, embracing the importance of Plan B means designing protocols that are robust to errors of individual components, involve failsafe measures and backup plans, and anticipate that parts will wear out and need replacement. The "Swiss cheese" model of error reduction is often used to describe medical systems that are resistant to failure and error. In this model each component is thought of as a slice of Swiss cheese with its own distribution of "holes" or vulnerabilities.[2] A properly designed system combines components in a way that offsets the holes of each part to minimizes the chances of an error propagating through the entire system. Conversely, a failure occurs when all the holes line up "just right."

Importantly, designing systems that absolutely require a particular step or subprocess to function in a very specific way is asking for potential failures. If you truly understand that every component could possibly fail—and every component certainly could—then you should take great care to not build protocols that ignore this fact.

As an example, during the very beginning of the COVID-19 pandemic in the United States, some initial triage protocols stated that they could 100 percent differentiate between patients with or without potential COVID-19 risk simply by asking if the patient had recently traveled to Wuhan, China. Even if we ignore for a moment the vast numbers of individuals who contracted the virus from person-to-person spread entirely outside of direct contact with individuals in China, this triage plan did not account for the fact that some individuals would not understand the question, might speak a different language, or might not answer the question truthfully. When a patient with a potential COVID-19 exposure was identified later in the emergency care process, there initially was often no effective Plan B in place to decrease collateral exposures. A more robust plan would have accounted for potential failure to appropriately triage at the initial junction, and provided a Plan B to isolate high-risk patients who were identified further along in the process.[3]

In summary, strong emergency responses result from combining individuals who proactively build and train Plan B methods directly into their approach, with systems that are designed to be robust to failure and resistant to error. In this way, you can build teams that resiliently address imperfection and maximize your chances for success.

Take Action

A useful way to identify and train alternative approaches that might be required if your primary protocols falter is to challenge yourself with mental simulations that start with failure—a process called a stumble-and-recovery drill. How would you respond if a particular tool you rely on was suddenly unavailable or if a commonly used process unexpectedly failed? What other systems would fail as a result, and what would be resilient to failure? How would you recover to achieve the objective?

Returning to the example of placing a breathing tube in this patient suffering from an allergic reaction, imagining realistic failures—such as the patient's airway being farther forward than expected or the light going out on the intubating blade—would facilitate the creation of basic, highly functional backup plans. Imagining more extreme failures—such as the power going out in the entire hospital during an attempted intubation—could help generate rarer but more creative backup plans, like not placing the patient on a vent and simply using a BVM system instead.

You can perform the same kind of mental simulation when designing robust protocols as part of a team. Imagine a key component failing—a server burning out, a key assumption being invalid, or some other reason that the protocol does not function as intended. How will your team recover to achieve the goal? What backup resources or contingency plans do you have, or should you put in place? How capable are you and your team at using these alternative approaches? What training might you put in place now as a result?

See Also

02 | Become a Student of Sangfroid
13 | Eliminate Unnecessary Opportunities for Failure
20 | Rapidly Accept Reality

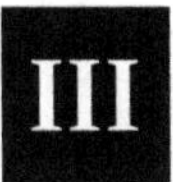

SUPPORTING
CRITICAL DECISIONS

11

MOVE FROM A TO B TO C

To improve rapid and effective performance when mental processing is at a premium, emergency providers use the ABC algorithm to structure their initial approach to critical, undifferentiated patients. ABC—airway, then breathing, then circulation—leverages the hierarchical dependencies inherent in human physiology to direct effort first to upstream problems before downstream issues are addressed. In this way, problems are confronted in efficient order and available resources are leveraged and maximized.

In the middle of a busy shift, the charge nurse comes over with news of a sick patient incoming, ETA two minutes. He's a young man who suffered a motorcycle crash at high speeds. The paramedics radioed in that he has difficulty breathing, multiple obvious broken bones, and a low blood pressure. According to the charge nurse, they seemed worried on the radio, which is an ominous sign.

The first time that you take the lead in a serious trauma case like this one, the scope of your job can easily feel overwhelming. Your patient might have multiple potential life-threatening injuries, there will be alarms going off around you, and everyone will be looking at *you* for direction and leadership. It can be easy to freeze, forget your training, and perform at a suboptimal level.

To structure your initial approach to a sick patient and bring order to the flow of the resuscitation even in chaotic situations, emergency providers utilize the ABC algorithm. ABC—which stands for airway, then breathing, then circulation—defines an order of operations that leverages core principles of human anatomy and physiology.

The strength of the ABC algorithm is that each step in the pipeline is a requirement for all subsequent steps to work: if step one (airway) is non-functional, then whether or not step two (breathing) is off-line or working properly is irrelevant. Since these sequential dependencies are inherent in human physiology, and therefore constant for all patients, solving problems in this order ensures that no effort is wasted and that patients get the best possible chance to survive their injuries.[1]

To understand how this works, let's do a rapid and simplified tour of cardiopulmonary anatomy and physiology in the context of this motorcycle accident. In order to keep this young man alive after his trauma, a primary goal is to make sure his brain gets oxygen. Without oxygen, his brain cells will starve and he will die. Oxygen is brought into the body via the lungs and transported to the brain via the circulatory system.

If your patient's blood is on the concrete after his accident, as opposed to inside his body where it should be, he has a circulatory problem. There might not be enough blood to transport the oxygen, or the pressure in his blood vessels might not be enough to push the blood to his brain.

However, if his lungs are not working—say because he suffered significant injuries to his chest during the accident—then his body would be unable to get oxygen from his lungs into his blood. In this case, he has a breathing problem. Even if his blood is inside him where it belongs, his body would still not be able to deliver oxygen to his brain.

Taking one further step back, if he had an airway problem, like significant facial or neck trauma, then he would be unable to get oxygen into his lungs in the first place. In this case, even if his lungs were working properly, there would be no oxygen arriving to put into the blood, and no oxygen to deliver to the brain.

Each step—A, then B, then C—must function properly before the next step has a chance to work. Knowing this, you can cut through the uncertainty and focus your energy where it is most needed by looking first at the airway, then progressing from there.

Importantly, the ABC algorithm is set up as a "do not pass go" strategy, meaning that if a problem is identified in one step, you do not move on to the next step until that problem is addressed. Additionally, if the patient's clinical status changes abruptly—if for example thirty minutes into the case his blood pressure drops un-expectedly—you should assume the scenario has changed and re-turn to the beginning of the ABC algorithm to plan your responses accordingly.

While not all crises have the same level of underlying strict dependencies like those powering the ABC algorithm, many types of emergencies do have some degree of hierarchical dependencies that can be used to help triage effort. For example, imagine you need to drive a friend to a hospital in a city without paramedic services. Getting your car started is initially more important than consulting any map or GPS system. Directions to the hospital are crucial, of course. But if your car doesn't start, then you'll need to focus first on getting other transportation; without transportation, the maps are irrelevant.

The more you know about the dependencies that exist in the situations in which you'll be acting, the better prepared you will be to leverage the correct order of operations and deploy your skills where they're most needed. Therefore, studying your craft not only as sets of individual facts or techniques, but also with an eye toward understanding the connections and hierarchies among concepts is vitally important as you build your emergency mind.

Take Action

Start by looking for sets of dependencies like "airway, breathing, circulation" throughout your field of practice. Where there are well-established dependencies with dedicated response algorithms like ABC, you can use these dependencies to help focus your training efforts.[2] If you know that Y depends on X, then you can concentrate on studying X before moving on to study Y. Otherwise, you might end up skilled at Y but unable to deploy that skill since your response would never make it past X.[3]

Where sets of dependencies are not well established, you can start to sketch out and test potential hierarchies. To generate ideas, look for both strict dependencies as well as functional dependencies. If the situation you're training for repeats over time, you can experiment by assuming different sets of dependencies to fine tune your understanding and performance. Eventually, you could consider developing algorithms to leverage what you find.

Before an event, use simulation or mental visualization to practice deploying your skills based on established or hypothesized sets of dependencies. If a crisis is likely to involve multiple different groups—like multiple teams responding to a large wildfire—you can use group walk-throughs or table-top exercises to practice and optimize responses. After an event, debriefs should identify and address any deviation from strict dependency-based algorithms, and evaluate the utility of following or modifying approaches to algorithms based on functional dependencies.

See Also

13 | Eliminate Unnecessary Opportunities for Failure
15 | Find the Rate-Limiting Step
25 | Use Algorithmic and Creative Thinking

12

LEARN TO ASK BETTER QUESTIONS

Your ability to respond effectively to a crisis is tied closely to the strength and quality of the questions you ask. Powerful questions will help you and your team move forward, while disempowering questions siphon energy and waste resources. The best questions during a crisis are present-focused and action-oriented. These questions are asked from within your sphere of influence and designed to address the most important decisions first.

Imagine two different sports teams debriefing in their respective locker rooms during halftime. In a pair of challenging and important games, both teams find themselves significantly behind, not having played up to their potential. As the athletes hydrate and stretch, their captains start to dig into what happened and what to do next.

The captain of one team opens the "discussion" with a series of heated questions: "What is wrong with you losers? What were you even thinking out there? How are we possibly going to recover and stop embarrassing ourselves?"

Across town in the locker room where the other group sits, the team captain asks a different set of questions: "How can we adjust right now to improve our performance in the second half? We're struggling out there. Remind me, what are we playing for? Who are we as a team? When you get back out there, what are each of you going to do differently?"

When they get back on the field, which team do you think has the better shot at rebounding from the first half and improving their performance? What about the next week at practice—which team would likely do a better job learning from their mistakes and avoiding further errors? Which set of questions is more likely to yield better answers? If they played each other later in the season, which team would you bet on?

Clearly, the second team has the chance to answer more useful questions in this scenario. As a result, the lessons these two teams learn will diverge considerably. The choices they make, how they train, and their performance in future engagements will all be affected by their leaders' choices regarding how to ask questions.

The same is true for you and your team, whether your arena is the athletic field or the emergency department. To improve your ability to perform under pressure, you need to learn to ask better questions. The differences between the questions you might ask are rarely as stark as the example above. You probably already know that yelling at someone (or being yelled at) never creates optimal conditions for learning. Still, taking the time to define what makes truly great questions—and then deliberately and consistently asking them—can drastically improve your opportunity to make better decisions.

So, what defines good questions to ask during a crisis? In this section we consider three key components of high-quality questions that hold up under conditions of uncertainty, pressure, and high potential impact.

First, the questions you ask in an emergency need to be focused on the right period of time. During an active event, this typically means that your questions should be exclusively present- and future-focused.

For example, during one particularly challenging case when I was struggling to secure a patient's airway, I opened an emergency cricothyrotomy kit only to find that the kit was missing several crucial components. It was an incredibly tense moment, and my patient's life hung in the balance. It would have been easy to ask past-focused questions—questions about who had stocked that kit or what could possibly explain why the components were missing. It also would have been useless. Asking those types of questions would have sucked energy and resources away from my team's attempts to resuscitate the patient in front of us. Instead, we needed to ask questions that were present-focused, questions about how we could use the components we did have to secure the patient's airway.[1]

Once you've safely completed your emergency response, then your questions can expand to consider both prior and future domains. After-action debriefs and focused learning should of course incorporate past-focused questions to figure out what happened and what you can do better in the future. Root-cause analyses, morbidity and mortality conferences, and other formal post hoc structures are extremely useful in transforming your experiences into improvements in future emergency responses. Taking care to focus your questions on the appropriate time frame will help you and your team operate at your highest possible ability and not divert scarce resources away from the critical problems in front of you.

Second, effective questions during an emergency need to be focused within your locus of control, and they need to be action oriented. Questions focused on parts of the situation where you have no ability to act—things outside your control—can be wasteful or dangerous during a crisis. Similarly, asking questions that are purely theoretical or will not change your response in this moment are generally inappropriate when you and your team are under significant pressure. Questions that are high-quality in this domain therefore tend to follow the structure of, "What can I do right now with what I have to best move myself and my team forward?"[2]

During a recent shift in the emergency department, for example, my team and I received an alert that our department would likely lose power in the next few moments. Monitors, elevators, computers—everything was going to shut down. We were in the middle of a trauma resuscitation and had several more incoming; it was clear this situation could present a significant challenge.

People immediately started shouting questions about why the power was going out, who would be held accountable, or what the city was going to do to get the power back on. Those questions, while absolutely understandable reactions, were not high-quality because they all focused on areas in which we had no control. Even if we had the head of the Department of Water and Power in the resuscitation room with us, able to provide expert-level answers to those particular questions, having those answers would not have improved our ability to actually respond to the emergencies at hand.

So, I reminded the team that while we didn't control the power, we did control our reaction to its loss, and we do control what questions we asked next.[3] Within a few moments, we were back to internally focused, action-oriented questions such as "What can we do in the next few minutes to organize paper charting systems for each patient? How do we ensure battery back-up power is available to key equipment?" Those questions were significantly better. They directed our collective attention to where it was most useful and encouraged answers that were actionable: What do we have the ability to change and how do we do that now?

Finally, the questions you ask during an emergency response should be tuned to address the most important, highest impact items first. Even if they are present-focused and action oriented, questions that address unimportant issues are not good questions. Since the compressed time frames mean you might only have the time to ask a very small number of questions during a emergency, devoting your attention to the most impactful decisions first ensures an effective order of operations.

The sequential survey system used in advanced trauma life support (ATLS) provides an important example of ordering questions based on their potential impact. In ATLS, the primary survey seeks to identify and address any immediately life-threatening issues, including critical abnormalities in the patient's airway, breathing, or circulation. This technique intentionally ignores injuries that are not immediately life-threatening—for example a sprained arm or minor abrasions—in favor of focusing on a limited number of crucial checkpoints.

The secondary survey by comparison seeks to catalogue and prioritize in order of importance every injury or issue a patient presents with. The secondary survey is exploratory in nature: it is broad, exhaustive, and tuned to not miss anything. Your goal with the secondary survey is to completely examine the patient, determine the extent of all injuries, and develop a plan for further work-up and treatment.

Importantly, if the patient's clinical condition changes at any point during the examination, you immediately start back over with the primary survey. In this way, you continually tune your focus and optimize your efforts to preferentially address life-threatening injuries or issues.

To summarize, effective questions are focused on what is happening right now and what you and your team can do about it. They are tuned to address the most important issues first, and as conditions change, so do they.

Take Action

Questioning your questions is a meta-cognitive skill that is easy to pick up and can yield significant benefits. You can start simply by watching the questions you ask and reflecting on their utility to your performance. Based on the criteria above, are you asking good questions when you find yourself in a crisis? What happens to these questions when the levels of pressure, uncertainty, and potential impact increase? Do your questions evolve and improve to keep pace, or do they break down in predictable ways?

If you find patterns where your questions could be better—for example being more present-focused during high-stress situations—begin practicing by asking these better questions in lower-stress environments. You could try writing down some strong questions ahead of a shift and seeing if you can use them in the flow of your work. Brainstorming with your peers about how and when to ask powerful questions can also yield excellent results.

Especially when you are new in a role, observing how more skilled providers ask questions is extremely useful. What types of questions are those in more senior roles asking, and why are they asking them? Thoughtful and self-reflective leaders should be able to discuss the quality of the questions they chose to ask after a hard case is over. A useful way to start this conversation with more experienced providers would be to find out what questions they routinely ask themselves now while responding to a crisis that they did not ask when they first started working on their craft. Ask for specific anecdotes or cases where high-quality questions made a difference in performance.

See Also

13

ELIMINATE UNNECESSARY OPPORTUNITIES FOR FAILURE

Unnecessary opportunities for failure are errors that you should be able to avoid or mitigate. Internal errors of this type occur when individuals make choices which unnecessarily diminish their ability to perform. External errors occur when systems or protocols contain potential points of failure that could easily have been addressed. Finding and eliminating these opportunities for failure is crucial to improving performance under pressure.

It was a challenging case and a complicated resuscitation. The patient—an elderly woman with multiple medical problems—arrived at your emergency department extremely ill and in septic shock from a complicated pneumonia. Her heart was racing, her blood pressure and oxygen were both dangerously low, and multiple organ systems appeared to be failing.

Placing a breathing tube without pushing her farther off into the physiologic deep end was a bit like threading the eye of a needle while standing on a moving train, but you and your team succeeded. As her numbers start to improve on the ventilator, you finally take a deep breath and reflect that it had really been a close call. Your relief, however, is short lived. As your team starts to move the patient to the intensive care unit, the ventilator begins to alarm, and her oxygen level again drops precipitously.

Running through the relevant algorithms, you identify the culprit. It's not a worsening of her disease process, nor is it a problem with your team's skillful resuscitation. She's not suffering because her medical needs are so complicated. Instead, the issue is something extremely simple, something that could have easily been avoided. The oxygen tank under her bed was empty, and no one had noticed.

Unfortunately, this scenario is all too real. Even the highest quality work of a skilled team can be brought down by this type of simple, avoidable mistake. This is a type of error you should be able to prevent or at least control—a category of error that emergency physician and Navy Lieutenant Commander Amy Hildreth, MD, calls an "unnecessary opportunity for failure."[1]

Not checking the level on the oxygen tank before transporting an oxygen-dependent patient is an unnecessary opportunity for failure. Unless the entire hospital is out of oxygen, this type of error did not have to happen. You and your team easily could have identified it ahead of time and addressed it before moving the patient.

Unnecessary opportunities for failure fall into two categories—internal and external—based on whether they are related to individual- or systems-level performance. Internal opportunities for failure include avoidable actions that diminish your ability to think clearly and perform at your best, such as failing to take care of yourself with proper nutrition, sleep, hydration, and exercise. An airline pilot sacrificing needed sleep and choosing to stay out late drinking before an early morning flight the next day would be choosing an unnecessary internal opportunity for failure. Showing up to the airport for the morning flight intoxicated would be an extreme (and unconscionable) example.

External opportunities for failure result from poorly designed or thoughtlessly executed structural or systemic factors that exist outside any individual team member. For example, emergency physician Chris Taicher, MD, tells the story of needing a particular piece of life-saving equipment for a critical patient he was treating during a night shift. Almost unbelievably, the item was stored in a locked room to which no one on the night shift had a key. The frustration he describes at being able to see the equipment through a window but not having access is both justified and palpable. Thankfully, his team was able to come up with an alternative solution, and his patient had a good outcome.[2]

The decision to lock the door to a critical equipment room is not necessarily a bad one—access to some types of equipment often does need to be restricted. But not thinking ahead to make sure the equipment could be accessed during all hours is an unnecessary external opportunity for failure. Returning to our initial example, the same might be said of not having a protocol for checking all vital components (such as the oxygen tank) related to an intubated patient before transporting that patient from the ER to the ICU. In both cases, these small structural factors could easily have led to catastrophic failures.

Any well-functioning team must make it a priority to find and mitigate unnecessary opportunities for failure. Unfortunately, they are often easiest to identify retrospectively after a loss or a suboptimal outcome.

When you, your team, or your system failed unnecessarily, you need to study what happened. You should deploy whatever solutions are necessary as soon as possible to prevent a repeat failure. In fact, not regularly reviewing your performance and looking for ways to improve your emergency response is—in and of itself—one of the most significant unnecessary opportunities for failure and a distinct waste of suffering.

Ideally, you would be able to identify unnecessary opportunities for failure before they occur. Two related techniques that individuals and teams can use to practice this are the Stoic philosophy concept of *premeditatio malorum* and the more modern technique of a premortem evaluation.

These two techniques are low-cost, easy to implement, and can be combined or used individually. Both techniques use mental visualization or simulation to "walk through" a process and identify areas that need to be addressed, and both can be rehearsed in low-pressure environments before being transitioned to use during a crisis.

Premeditatio malorum translates roughly from Latin as "thinking ahead about evils." To employ this tactic—which is also known as negative visualization—you mentally walk through a case or procedure from the beginning and visualize every possible failure along the way.[3]

If you were designing a better protocol for transporting patients on ventilators from the emergency department to the intensive care unit, you could utilize *premeditatio malorum* to brainstorm every possible way that anything could break or falter, and every way that your team could stumble.

Your resulting long list would probably include items such as the power failing on the ventilator battery, the elevator getting stuck while you were in it, or the patient needing more sedation or blood pressure medication urgently while you were en route. Your team could respond with either ad hoc solutions, such as carrying a backup battery, or more systemic responses, like developing a protocol that included double checking the transport route before starting to roll.

In a premortem evaluation, you work in the other direction, using mental visualization to imagine a universe in which the process you're attempting is over, and, unfortunately, you failed. Starting from that assumed failure, you mentally work backward to figure out how and why things went wrong. Paraphrasing the Nobel prize-winning psychologist-economist Daniel Kahneman, mentally moving backward like this disrupts the normal assumptions you might make and allows you more freedom of thought and creativity to identify problems and potential solutions.[3]

To continue the ICU transport example, prior to moving the patient, you might gather the transport team together, explain the exercise, and imagine as a group the unfortunate scenario where the patient died as you were traveling to the ICU. What went wrong, and what could you have done about it?

Starting from the end like this might reveal problems such as the intensive care team not being ready to receive the patient, the breathing tube becoming dislodged as you physically transferred the patient to the unit bed, or a crucial resource like oxygen running out before you reached your destination. Each way that you can visualize failure becomes a chance to design and implement a solution—one that minimizes the probability of the imagined failure becoming reality.

Certainly, not everything that goes wrong during an emergency is an "unnecessary" failure. In fact, there are an infinite number of ways in which something can go unpredictably or uncontrollably wrong during a crisis. You cannot possibly identify or plan ahead for all of them.

What you can do though, is make sure you consciously seek out and address unnecessary opportunities for failure in your particular work environment. After all, there are plenty of "smart" ways out there for a project to fail or a system to break. There is absolutely no need for "dumb" causes that could have been avoided.

Take Action

At a basic level, eliminating unnecessary opportunities for failure is about leveraging thinking before an emergency to improve your chances of making good decisions during the emergency. The best way to start employing this mental model is during the downtime between active emergency responses.

You can start by considering a few of the most common critical moments in your environment—such as placing a breathing tube or transporting a severely ill patient—when the stakes are particularly high. Pick one of these moments, and perform a premortem evaluation or use negative visualization, looking for sources of potential failure. Doing this exercise in a group is often helpful, since different types of operators will have different vantage points on what is likely to fail and why.

When you have several options for potential sources of failure, consider which ones might be addressed ahead of time, and get to work fixing them. Proactively addressing unnecessary opportunities for failure should be celebrated publicly to help make looking for these errors a larger part of your team's culture.

If you are more junior and can't quite visualize a particular process yet or otherwise don't know where to start, you can begin by considering a recent challenging case and analyzing that case backward. Consider asking individuals who were involved how they think the case could have gone better, or what they now wish they had known earlier. When you find examples of unnecessary opportunities for failure, look laterally to where else that error might be lurking. For example, if you realize that transports from the emergency department to the ICU should include a check of the backup oxygen tank, what other instances of patient transport might need to be checked?

See Also

05 | Train Your Tired Moves
16 | Commit to Never Waste Suffering
22 | Find Your Locus of Control

14

DECIDE TO NOT DECIDE

The number of decisions you face during a crisis can easily become overwhelming. Thankfully, you don't have to make every decision. Decisions that are easily reversible, have low impact, or do not address the primary forces at play can often be safely ignored or deferred. Rapidly identifying which decisions you do not need to make will help you focus energy on those that definitely need your attention.

To effectively respond to a crisis, it's not enough to just make decisions correctly; you need to make the *correct* decisions correctly. Not all decisions during a crisis are equally important, and your focus and energy are finite resources. So, you need to make sure you're devoting your attention to the most important decisions, not just whatever decisions you happen to be faced with at that moment.

As an example, imagine you are the founder of a relatively young company and you're scheduled to give an important demo in an hour. If you impress your audience, you are likely to land a lucrative contract. If you fail, your team will run out of money within the week, and you might have to close shop. Sitting in your hotel room, you get two emails. The first is from your head engineer, warning that she just found a critical failure in the product you're planning to show. The second is from your sales manager asking for direction on prioritizing between two potential client meetings next month.

In this moment, there are a variety of decisions you could make. Do you believe the assessment of your engineer? Should you cancel the demo or proceed anyway? If you do proceed, what should you change to account for the new information? Over the next few months, how much time should your sales team spend on different categories of clients?

Clearly, not all these decisions are equally relevant, even though they all arrived at the same moment. Deciding between going forward with the demo or canceling is probably critically important to the future of your company. Planning details around the next quarter's sales strategy is not nearly as urgent. In fact, even a "perfect" decision regarding long-term sales strategies will not help you or your team respond to the problem you're currently facing.

To perform well under pressure, you must be able to identify those decisions that require your immediate attention. But it is equally important to identify your least critical decisions and have the discipline to put those aside.

During an emergency, the most critical decisions are those that irreversibly (or at least strongly) commit your team to a particular mental model or course of action. These decisions involve high-stakes outcomes and can drastically influence subsequent downstream options. Conversely, decisions that can be easily and cheaply reversed with minimal potential impact, or those that are extremely limited in the scope of their influence, are generally less important.

To explore these differences, let's consider two decisions emergency physicians are called to make when caring for someone suffering from an acute stroke: the decision to deliver a thrombolytic ("clot-busting") medication to try to open up blocked blood vessels in the brain, and the decision to use a calcium channel blocker (CCB) drip to control the patient's blood pressure.

Determining whether or not to give a patient thrombolytics is typically considered to be the single most important decision during an acute stroke case. If the medication works, it allows blood to once again reach the injured areas of the patient's brain. In this case, the patient's symptoms can improve markedly or even resolve completely. However, the medication also has significant potential side effects and can cause life-threatening bleeding or even death. Obviously, this decision has high potential impact.

Additionally, once thrombolytics are delivered, they cannot be turned off, and they cannot be reversed. Deciding to use thrombolytics commits your team to a single course of action. Many other subsequent decisions—including otherwise simple choices like whether or not to place an IV line—become complicated risk-benefit calculations after thrombolytics have been used. So, this one decision also impacts future downstream choices.

Using a CCB drip to control a patient's blood pressure during an acute stroke is a very different type of decision. While blood-pressure control is certainly important during a stroke, precise control is often not significantly better than slightly looser control. In fact, you sometimes allow blood pressure to ride higher than normal in an attempt to support the brain in perfusing blood past a blockage.

As such, the relative impact of this decision is much less significant than whether or not to give thrombolytics.

Unlike thrombolytics, CCB drips are titratable and can be easily adjusted up or down, or even rapidly turned off. This decision is therefore cheaply reversible with limited long-term effects and does not typically commit your team to a single course of action. Finally, most other decisions about caring for a patient with an acute stroke are not impacted by whether or not CCBs are used.

Choosing whether or not to use a CCB drip to control your patient's blood pressure is an important decision in many situations. But in this particular case, it is much less critical than your decision concerning thrombolytics. As a result, you should put much more of your energy into deciding whether or not to give thrombolytics than CCBs.[1]

One crucial way to identify low-importance decisions is to look for equipoise, which refers to the situation where there is little to no difference in the expected outcomes between options in a decision. Equipoise might be reached because the different options you are considering have largely similar results. For example, if you are deciding between two antibiotics, both with expected success rates of 90 percent for a given type of infection, there is equipoise between the antibiotic choices. Alternatively, equipoise might be reached because you genuinely do not know which option will yield a better outcome, for example when the best available evidence disagrees about the utility of a given treatment.

When you identify equipoise in a decision, you should strongly consider not devoting further energy to it, and instead investing that energy somewhere else. Additional time spent studying the decision is unlikely to make a significant impact in the outcome. To conserve decision-making energy in these cases you could choose between the options randomly, or you could utilize "intelligent defaults." Those defaults would suggest a choice based on outside criteria, such as which antibiotic is in greater supply in your pharmacy at the moment. Alternatively, you could rely on general principles such as "first, do no harm," and default to not offering a treatment when evidence is conflicting.

An important concept related to equipoise is "freerolling," which applies to a situation in which such an asymmetry exists between the upside and downside of a certain choice that the decision becomes almost unnecessary.[2] For example, one potential cause of cardiac arrest is hypoglycemia (low blood sugar), the treatment for which is administration of glucose (sugar). So, one plan of action during a cardiac arrest would be to test the patient's blood glucose level and give extra glucose only if needed. However, if the patient's glucose level is normal or even high, giving extra glucose during a cardiac arrest actually will not cause any adverse effects. Because there is no downside and considerable potential upside, the decision whether or not to give the glucose is—in this specific situation—a freeroll. As a result, you might choose to just give the glucose before the test result is back and move on to make other, more impactful decisions.

We've discussed that not all decisions are equally important. But it is also true that you cannot make every decision well. The faster you identify which decisions you do not have to make and decide to not make them, the more time and energy you can spend on the choices that matter the most. As martial arts legend Bruce Lee famously said, "It is not daily increase but daily decrease, hack away the unessential."

Take Action

When you are just starting to practice your craft—or when you find yourself performing in unfamiliar circumstances—it can be challenging to identify which decisions are the most important ones to make and which ones can safely receive less attention. When your level of expertise is low, every choice can feel critically important since the implications of the choices are not yet clear to you. It's a good idea to speak to more experienced providers during an off period and ask them how they divide their energy differently now than when they started out. If you have a series of decisions to make, ask them which they identify as the most important.

It is particularly useful to observe more senior operators when they do not make a decision that you anticipated and thought would be important. After the crisis is over, ask them to walk you through the logic of not making that particular decision. Their answer could reveal implicit assumptions, or parts of a mental model, of which you were not aware.

As a more senior provider, try to explicitly state when you are choosing not to make a decision and why (if time allows), as that information can be extremely helpful for junior learners. Additionally, self-reflection on what decisions you think are the most important during a particular emergency—either through post hoc recall or through decision notes you take in the moment—can help you identify and evaluate unconscious patterns in your own thinking.

Finally, both junior and senior operators can benefit from running through simulated or table-top cases in group settings while explicitly talking about their decision making. Discussing why someone chose to make a particular decision, not just how, can help you identify the logic your peers use and provide suggestions for potential improvement.

See Also

15

FIND THE RATE-LIMITING STEP

The rate-limiting step of a process is the slowest part of its execution. Identifying the rate-limiting step is critical to effective decision making under pressure, since this step acts as a choke on the speed of your overall progress. Often, the rate-limiting step is not the most technically or theoretically complex part of a process, but something mundane or easily overlooked. When the rate-limiting step cannot be easily determined, you should take this as a signal to invest more energy in understanding the details of the emergency you're facing and your potential actions.

In a chemical reaction, whichever part is the slowest dictates the overall speed with which the whole reaction can take place. This step—called the rate-limiting step or the rate-determining step—might not be the most complicated part of the process or the most energy intensive, but it nevertheless sets the pace. As a result, modifying the speed at which this particular step proceeds will significantly change the kinetics of the entire reaction.[1]

Similarly, the rate-limiting step in an emergency situation is the process that takes the longest to accomplish while addressing a particular crisis. It is not necessarily the most technically complicated or difficult-to-perform part of the process; it is just the part that takes the longest to accomplish and, thus, prevents other parts from actively moving forward.

When you've identified the rate-limiting step during an emergency, you can make decisions that effectively prioritize individual and team actions despite high pressure and uncertainty. When it is not identified, your plans will be inefficient at best and potentially even non-functional or counterproductive.

Consider the rate-limiting step in delivering an electric shock to your patient during a cardiac arrest. A great deal of thought and training goes into identifying cardiac rhythms that would benefit from electrical shocks. For example, to become certified in advanced cardiac life support, you must prove that you understand how and when to use a defibrillator in various situations during a cardiac arrest.

Despite all of this sophisticated training, the rate-limiting step in delivering a successful electric shock is typically not related to executing a complex decision algorithm, nor is it identifying the sometimes-subtle differences in electrical activity in various types of cardiac arrest. The rate-limiting step is often something much more mundane—rolling the patient over to expose the back.

Let's explore why. Cardiac defibrillators deliver electricity to a patient's heart by passing current between two electrode pads. In most modern systems, one pad is placed in the center of the patient's chest, and the other in the center of the back. Placing a pad on the patient's chest is easy, but until your team is able to place the electrode pad on the patient's back, the defibrillator cannot deliver electrical current to the heart.[2]

Rolling the patient over to place the electrode pad therefore becomes a key rate-limiting step in effective cardiac arrest care. No matter how well trained your team is, you cannot deliver a shock without positioning that second electrode pad. Teams that recognize the reality of this rate-limiting step will roll patients earlier in their resuscitation to prioritize placing an electrode pad. As a result, they likely will be able to deliver electricity much earlier than teams that ignore or neglect this "simple" step.

As this example shows, rapidly and accurately identifying the rate-limiting step in responding to an emergency is critical to effective performance. So how do you identify those steps?

Some emergencies are well understood, and the steps it takes to best respond to them are mapped out and easy to process.[3] For situations that fall into this category—such as delivering an electrical shock during a cardiac arrest—you can usually successfully identify the rate-limiting step by mentally or experimentally moving through the process, and simply measuring what takes the most time or effort to accomplish.

For example, using a fiber-optic camera to place a breathing tube requires a well-known series of steps. Running repetitions of simulated cases that require this technique can help you identify the rate-limiting step in assembling your tools, preparing the patient, and securing the airway. After identifying this step—typically getting the camera up and running—protocols could be tuned to preferentially focus on the relevant issue, or engineering solutions could be attempted to speed the step up, thereby improving the entire emergency response.

Other emergencies have less predictable structures, or may involve components with multiple or non-linear inputs that can complicate identification of the rate-limiting step. Consider a patient who presents to the emergency department with potential meningitis, an infection of the space around the brain that can be life threatening and highly contagious. To diagnose meningitis, you would typically perform a CT scan of the head, followed by a lumbar puncture to obtain cerebrospinal fluid for analysis.

Depending on the day and load on the system from other patients, the rate-limiting step in this process can vary widely. Perhaps it's a busy time in your department, with many other patients who also require CT imaging. In that case, the slowest step for this patient could be obtaining a CT scan. Perhaps the most time-consuming step is performing the lumbar puncture, which can sometimes be quite technically challenging or require sedation. Alternatively, perhaps the slowest step is something more mundane, like finding the lumbar-puncture kit in the stockroom or physically transporting the patient to the CT scanner. In this case, Identifying the rate-limiting step may involve gathering data on the flow of information and patients through other areas of your department or assessing the load on shared resources such as the CT scanner.

Unlike in a chemical reaction where the rate-limiting step will always be the same given the same reagents, the rate-limiting step across multiple repetitions of even nearly identical emergencies might vary widely and might require unique investigation in each instance. Whatever the rate-limiting step is, identifying it is the first step toward overcoming barriers to treating your patient and designing systems that can better respond to crises.

Returning to the example of the patient with potential meningitis, knowing the rate-limiting step might allow you to optimize different risk-benefit decisions. Meningitis needs to be treated rapidly, and if you believe the diagnosis might take a few hours by the time the lab reports back, you might choose to deliver antibiotic therapy empirically, even in the absence of complete proof of the diagnosis.

At the department level, if you know a patient will be occupied for a period of time getting a CT scan, you can more effectively deploy your attention elsewhere and advance the care of other patients. You might not be able to change the speed at which a CT happens, but you can change the way your team deploys resources as a result. Alternatively, if you routinely find that the rate-limiting step is structural—such as not knowing the location of the lumbar-puncture kit—you can implement systems-level changes such as changing the kits' location in the stockroom.

As a final note, as the situation in an emergency changes, so, too, does the rate-limiting step of your response. The better you understand the barriers to optimally responding to an emergency, the faster you can respond and the more effective your response will be. That said, constantly chasing a changing rate-limiting step can be as inefficient as not knowing it in the first place; you need to effectively divide your resources between studying a problem and executing a solution.

Take Action

A simple way to start working with the concept of finding the rate-limiting step during a crisis is to pause briefly, when it is safe to do so, and ask yourself what is preventing you from making progress. Once you have an idea of what needs to be accomplished, work backward from there to try to identify what slowest step in the chain is between where you are now and where you want to be. Assuming you have a good handle on the situation, you've just found the rate-limiting step and can now get to work addressing it.

If you're simultaneously managing multiple emergencies, you can scale this idea up by quickly running through each scenario and identifying the set of rate-limiting steps. Then, among these rate-limiting steps, think about which will be the slowest or have the greatest impact on the whole set. Whatever you identify, that's where you should spend your decision-making energy.

In the emergency department, this is called "running the board"—periodically looking briefly through every active case in the department and identifying its rate-limiting step. The repetition of this approach also helps you identify those patients for whom you're still missing the rate-limiting step—meaning that you don't yet have a good understanding of the patient's underlying problem or treatment.

Finally, if resources permit and you're interested in improving your performance at a particular skill—say placing a central line or using the fiber-optic intubating camera—consider actually timing the steps and empirically identifying your own rate-limiting step. Once you identify that, what could you and your team do to improve your performance on that one skill?

See Also

11 | Move from A to B to C
21 | See the Forest and the Leaf
24 | Combine Action and Analysis

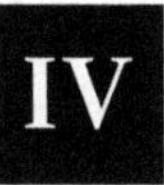

BUILDING FROM
CORE VALUES

16

COMMIT TO NEVER WASTE SUFFERING

No matter how skilled you become at performing under pressure, you cannot stop all suffering. You can, however, build and grow from that suffering. Committing to never wasting suffering means that you choose to leverage your experiences and those of your patients to improve yourself and your team and to learn to provide better care for your next patient. It means choosing to see suffering not as the end of a process, but as fuel for change and learning.

Suffering is a part of life. What you choose to do with that suffering—how you respond to it, process it, and transform it—has significant implications in both your day-to-day existence and in your ability to respond during a crisis. In fact, when I think of everything I've learned during my time as an emergency physician and everything I've put into The Emergency Mind project, perhaps the single most important lesson is this: never waste suffering.

Never waste the suffering your patients experience, and never waste your own.

To waste suffering is to allow poor outcomes to happen without learning from them. It is to believe that nothing could be changed or improved at the end of a hard case, either internally or externally, to better prepare you and your team for tomorrow's emergencies. In a sense, it is to be defeated, to give up.

By comparison, when you resolve to never waste your patients' suffering or your own, you commit to learn from everything that happens. Rather than be crushed by what happened, you choose to leverage today's issues to perform better tomorrow and every day thereafter. If you want to get better at performing under pressure, you cannot waste suffering. It is too precious a resource.

Structurally, wasting suffering tends to take two forms, either internalizing it or externalizing it. Both of these are equally futile responses and neither functions to push you or your team forward.

Some individuals waste suffering by holding onto it too tightly or internalizing it too much. In this case, you are overly focused on how poorly you might have performed, or you beat yourself up over the result without working to draw lessons from what happened. Often, this path spirals quickly to self-defeating generalizations about how awful you are at your craft or what a terrible person you are. This lowered self-confidence can easily result in impostor syndrome or poor performance during subsequent crises.

Alternatively, individuals might waste suffering by running away from it or over-externalizing it. In this case, instead of looking into what you could learn, you focus on everything outside your control that contributed to the recent poor outcome. You might blame equipment, teammates, environmental factors, or anything else to shift the focus away from actually figuring out what happened. Often, this path leads to frustrated, angry responses, friction and tension among teammates, and, again, poor performance in subsequent emergencies.

When you commit to never wasting suffering, you take a pledge to yourself, your teams, and the individuals you serve. In doing so, you commit to consistently leverage your experiences, to seek growth over comfort, and to use everything you are given to get better at what you do. Often this work is invisible and internal. It is the day-to-day grind of hammering on your craft and choosing to seek the marginal gains it takes to improve yourself.[1] Personally, when this feels particularly challenging, I reinforce my commitment by saying out loud to myself, "I will not waste this suffering."

You can learn this lesson outside the emergency department as well. For example, in jiu-jitsu when you're submitted or lose a match, you experience the mental suffering of having made a mistake and often the physical suffering of being caught in a painful lock. Each time this happens, you can choose how to process that suffering, to honor or ignore your commitment to never waste it.[2] By accepting what happened and asking yourself with a non-judgmental mind how you might perform better next time, you can transform that suffering into growth.

You might, for example, attempt to recreate the situation just prior to failure and run drills from that position, or discuss with your opponent or partner what weakness they found in your strategy that you could improve. However you choose to do it, honoring your commitment to never waste suffering means taking that loss or failure not as an end point, but as the beginning of what comes next. Yes, it is still suffering and yes it is hard and painful, but it is also an opportunity to improve and further master your craft.

Externally, committing to never waste suffering means first that you and your team must be able to talk about suffering. That commitment must become part of your culture. On the simplest level, you can remind your team about your choice and make it part of your daily work; ask each other what you learned that day and what skill or process you plan to improve.

More formal structures might involve regular reviews of emergency responses with poor outcomes and team-based evaluation of any systemic problems. Root cause analyses, which seek to identify the primary underlying cause of a mistake or a bad outcome in a case, can be used to help process events and identify areas for individual and systemic improvement.[3]

For example, suppose your team had struggled to place a breathing tube during a challenging case in the emergency department. Your primary equipment had malfunctioned, and, for whatever reason, your backup equipment was more difficult to access than you had anticipated.

Honoring your commitment to never waste suffering, you might reflect on the case using a team debrief, and collectively discuss what you learned about yourselves and your systems from your struggles. Perhaps you could have improved your initial assessment of the patient's airway, predicted a difficult intubation, and consequently spent more time ensuring your backup tools were ready.

Rather than just be frustrated about the difficult-to-find backup equipment, you might choose to undertake a more formal analysis of your logistics and supply structures to better ask why your backup tools were hard to come by. Should you store it somewhere else? Train more individuals how to set it up? How can you make sure you will be better able to care for a similar patient tomorrow, the next day, and in five years?[4]

Crucially, working to never waste suffering does not mean that you ignore the reality of what you went through. You should never skip the internal processing. You need to handle the residue of your experiences.[5] You are human, and the suffering you'll experience as an emergency provider can hit you and your teammates very, very hard. Attempting to rush through the processing of your emotions and head directly into learning does not work. It is important and worthwhile to allow yourself the space and time you need to open up, process your experience, and sort out the full range of your feelings before working on systemic improvement.

Take Action

You will encounter many opportunities to leverage suffering. Some will come during an acute response to an emergency, and some will come during your day-to-day life. Once you've made the commitment to never waste suffering, start practicing that commitment with small levels of frustration, difficulty, or loss. If you lose a practice match on the jiu-jitsu mat or a game of chess against a friend, use that loss as an opportunity. Get curious about internal factors, such as how you mentally and physically respond to suffering, and external factors, like how you could have played better or understood deeper levels of the game. What does it feel like to commit to learning from the experience as opposed to running away from it?

If you engage in a repeated activity, like the long-term practice of an art or sport, it can be useful to keep a journal of what setbacks you encounter and what you learned from those setbacks. You might, for example, write down something you struggled with every session and what you did about it, or what you need to try next.

Similarly, at the end of an emergency, take a few moments to jot down what you experienced and what you learned or hope to learn from it. Whenever possible, participating in team debriefs after an event will not only help you better process your own suffering but also expose you to different models of how more senior providers leverage theirs.

See Also

02 | Become a Student of Sangfroid
06 | Practice *Wabi-Sabi*
22 | Find Your Locus of Control

17

HUMANS NOT ROBOTS

Being human during an emergency is not easy. In the short run, it can feel simpler to pretend to be a robot and ignore what you need, what you feel, and the residue that a crisis leaves with you. However, your humanity is not a weakness but a source of deep strength. Understanding how your body and mind prepare for and process stress and pressure will help you perform at your best, recover from difficult experiences, and return to strive again.

Performing in the crucible of an emergency can be dehumanizing. Even with significant experience and skill in responding to emergencies, you can lose sight of your deeper self or start to view the individuals around you more as mannequins or actors in a play than as other humans. As you work through the extreme pressure and unfamiliar situations, it is often tempting to ignore internal signals like emotions and physical sensations, and to miss the depth, character, and humanity of people around you.

Remembering that you, the people on your team, and the people you serve during a crisis are all human is a source of great strength and a crucial component of your emergency mind. Emergency physician Emily Brumfield, MD, put it this way as she described the challenge in learning to see herself as a human, not a robot, when performing under pressure, "I used to come to work and just try to 'robot' so hard. I didn't think of my humanness as an important part of my 'physician-ness'... now it feels like the only way I can take care of people is by being human."[1]

Honoring your humanity during an emergency involves several interconnected concepts. First, it means learning about fueling and taking care of your body and mind so you are capable and ready to respond to a crisis. Second, it means understanding that every person responds to an emergency differently, and that processing your personal response is part of your job. Third and finally, it means learning to recognize and address the often painfully deep stress that encountering trauma and crisis can place on you, your teammates, and the individuals you serve.

On a physical level, your ability to deploy your skills during a crisis depends on the state of your body and mind at the moment of that emergency. As someone who is training to perform under the pressure of an emergency situation, you are an athlete, and you need to treat yourself like one. Sleep and hydration are crucially important factors affecting human performance, as is the balance between energy intake and the mental and physical outputs required to perform your craft. *Your human system—your body and your mind—is just as important as any other system you work with.* Ignoring how it is optimally primed and maintained leads to decreased performance and suboptimal outcomes.[2]

A great example of proactively addressing the connection between taking care of your human system and your ability to perform under pressure comes from the aviation industry. One tool that pilots use to help ensure that they are physically and mentally prepared to fly an aircraft is the "I'M SAFE" self-evaluation checklist.[3] Undertaking an I'M SAFE evaluation requires pilots to examine themselves for signs of (I) illness, (M) medication effects, (S) stress, (A) alcohol, (F) fatigue, and (E) emotional upset before starting their flight. In some cases, the "E" of I'M SAFE is replaced with eating/elimination to make sure pilots also pay attention to their basic biological needs prior to take off. Monitoring these core pillars of human performance helps ensure that pilots have the necessary building blocks to safely perform their work. Any individual—pilot or not—could use this protocol to assess their own readiness prior to responding to a crisis.

Once a crisis has started, you need to remember that your patients and their family members are human beings, not just cases to attend to. Typically, your patients will not have specific training in how to perform under pressure. They might be scared or confused. Being ill can be terrifying and painful, as can seeing your loved ones suffering and hooked up to machines. Many individuals feel powerless as a result, especially those who are coming face to face with the reality of a serious illness or potential loss for the first time. As a result, they might express these feelings by lashing out in anger, shutting down in fear, or otherwise acting out.

Treating the terror, suffering, and grief of people involved in a crisis is just as much a part of your job in the emergency department as treating their illnesses and injuries. If they bring fear or anger into your department, you need to work to create safe spaces to buffer those feelings and try to offer compassion in return. What might be a totally routine process for you might also be the single worst day of someone else's life, or the first time an individual has considered the mortality of someone they love dearly.

There is, of course, a balance to this, and the way you bring your humanity to a crisis can vary. If your patient is dying on hospice care, then asking family members about what the person loves to do or what brings them joy might be the best medicine you could possibly deliver. However, for an individual in a car accident with a broken leg, asking about a childhood pet before providing pain medicine would be cruel. In the extreme example of a life-threatening tension pneumothorax—where air building up in the chest cavity is preventing the heart from beating—the most compassionate, human-to-human action you can take is to stab the patient in the chest with a large-bore needle in order to relieve the pressure.

After you go through difficult experiences such as the death of a patient or having made a crucial mistake, part of being human is processing what happened. This is not easy. However, ignoring what you feel after an event as opposed to addressing it—in effect, pretending to be a robot—leads to dysfunction and burnout. Learning to bring compassion to yourself and your teams is critically important, as are talking about the effects of trauma on your lives and working actively to process your emotions and reactions to difficult events.

A useful way to understand and address what happens after you go through an emergency is the concept of "residue." Put simply, difficult experiences leave residue that can build up and block or choke your system if you don't address it, just like the residue in a water pipe can build up and impede flow. Actor Tom Hardy, in discussion with the Mission Critical Teams Institute, describes residue as follows:

As an actor I immerse myself in a character. When the movie production is over and it is time for me to immerse myself in a new character, there is still remnants or residue of the previous character within me. I need to undertake a process to remove, absorb or accept that residue in order to prepare for the next character I will embody.[4]

Conceptualized in this way, processing residue is a natural part of experiencing an emergency, *not* a mark of weakness or a flaw. When you acknowledge the residue of an experience and begin to work with it, you set the stage for healing and growth. You also improve your desire and ability to come back in tomorrow and try again.

At the team or organizational level, you can support individuals in being humans and not robots first and foremost by expressing your own humanity, and by building a culture that expects humanity from the individuals around you. Celebrate choices that empower team members to show up for work ready to perform at their best, discuss residue directly, expect and honor the need to process it, and create supportive spaces for individuals experiencing trauma.

As a concrete example in the emergency department, you can support your team by taking a moment of silence after the death of patient. Certainly not all residue can be processed in the minute immediately after a patient passes. But by taking that quiet pause, you can normalize the need to feel things, open the door to your emotions however they might show up, honor the person who just passed, and acknowledge your shared humanity.

Take Action

While structures like the I'M SAFE protocol help you identify the minimum requirements for safe performance, it's a more complicated process to optimize your nutrition, sleep, hydration, and mental and physical exertion for emergency response. What works best for one person might not function at all for another. Learning how to best care for yourself as a human is an individual responsibility that typically requires experimentation, reflection, and tinkering.

An easy way to start this process is to take the advice of athlete, coach, and performance-science expert Kristen Holmes who says that what we choose to do on our *days off* deeply affects what we're able to do during our *days on*.[5] Start thinking about this relationship and how it functions for you personally. You might take notes on what you eat or how you exercise and rest during your days off and compare those notes to how well you function during your days on.

Personally, I find that daily exercise, consciously training gratitude, and engaging in meditation (or some sort of reflection practice) make enormous differences in my ability to be a good emergency physician. Even simple changes, like how much water you drink before starting a shift, can have disproportionately large impacts on your ability to perform during a crisis.

After an event, there is no universal prescription in terms of how to process the residue you might face. Recognizing residue when you experience it and naming it as an expected part of the emergency response is a big victory and an important place to start. Designating "residue-processing time" during your day or week when you journal or simply reflect can be useful. An even simpler but still powerful step would be to just say out loud, "I am feeling residue," when you notice it occurring.

Explaining the concept of residue to the people in your lives who are "civilians" and don't train to perform in crises can also help to open crucial lines of communication. The simple step of naming what you feel when you feel it can sometimes slow the "leak" of the stress you're processing into other areas of your life. Talking about processing residue with individuals more experienced in your craft or working with professional counselors are also key resources that can help you handle extreme experiences in productive—or at least non-harmful—ways.

See Also

02 | Become a Student of Sangfroid
07 | Understand Fallibility and Cognitive Bias
18 | Start from First Principles

18

START FROM FIRST PRINCIPLES

Your actions under pressure should at all times reflect your deepest values. The more clearly you understand these values, the easier it will be to make sure your choices align with who you and your team are and want to be. You must explore your ethical frameworks ahead of time, before a crisis. You can test these frameworks the same way you test your technical skills, by applying graduated pressure.

Imagine you are the emergency doctor at a small hospital. You are partway through your shift when the radio goes off with news of multiple casualties incoming. Nearby, a driver lost control of his car and flew head-on into a group of other cars, some of which then rolled down a steep embankment. The details are unclear, but in the next few minutes you are expecting multiple victims, several of whom have potentially life-threatening injuries requiring immediate attention.

Your facility simply does not have the resources it would need to simultaneously care for all these individuals, and your team is going to be overwhelmed. Knowing this, whom do you attend to first? How do you ration your limited resources? Which patient should get the most intensive care, and which patient might need to receive less?

In addition to the technical, mental, and interpersonal skills you need to deploy when responding to a crisis, emergencies will often require you to make trade-offs between the rights and needs of different individuals and communities. To help guide you in these complicated decisions, you need to leverage your personal ethical principles and those of your team and organization. These ideas are your core moral concepts; they help you define your deepest values as a human and serve as guideposts for your actions in difficult circumstances.

Thankfully, not all emergency situations involve ethical dilemmas. If you are slammed by a large wave while surfing and held underwater, you can concentrate on staying calm and controlling your oxygen consumption without needing to worry about other people also having enough to breathe. However, many emergencies *do* involve these complex, higher-order decisions and require you to look within yourself to understand what you believe and what type of person you want to be as you respond.

A fundamental principle in performing under pressure is that your actions should at all times reflect your deepest values. A corollary is that the better you personally understand your moral principles—the more clarity you have about your core beliefs—the more capable you'll be of acting in tune with these principles.

Like the other components of your emergency mind, your personal ethical frameworks need to be developed and practiced ahead of time before you are under significant pressure. It is unrealistic to expect that you could perform well during a crisis involving a significant ethical component after simply looking through a list of ethical tenets. Telling someone to "respect humanity" does not help that person understand how to accomplish that goal under pressure. Technical skills—like slowing down your breathing during a critical step of a procedure—require practice under conditions of graduated pressure, and the application of ethics to emergencies is no different. You need to explore your ethical principles early and often, typically through visualizing and debating actions in hypothetical cases and post hoc analyses of behaviors during actual crises.[1]

Within the world of emergency medicine (and the world of medicine in general) ethics is taught alongside anatomy and physiology during medical training. That's because it is fundamentally not possible to provide effective medical care without understanding the broader context within which medicine operates in humanity and in community life.

The core tenets of medical ethics are autonomy, justice, beneficence, and non-maleficence. Autonomy refers to the right of individuals to make decisions for themselves. Justice describes the principle of equal access to the burden and benefit of medical treatment. Beneficence explains that all treatment must be for the net benefit of the patient and the community. Finally, non-maleficence is the principle of minimizing harm to individuals and society. Collectively, these tenets give medical providers a framework within which potential decisions can be evaluated and compared. While acting ethically is always important during the provision of emergency medical care, ethics comes more to the forefront of the decision-making process when multiple principles need to be balanced against each other.

Consider for example, how you and your team might handle the following situation: one of the victims from the car crash seems to have suffered a serious head injury but refuses treatment and is attempting to get off the gurney and leave. How do you balance a desire to respect autonomy and his right to refuse care with the importance of non-maleficence, and not letting this patient harm himself further?

In this case, you would need to make a context-specific judgment by weighing these two moral principles against each other and try to determine which action is "most right." Typically, emergency providers in this circumstance would determine that the patient's head injuries prevent him from understanding the risks of his decision and, therefore, from competently exercising his autonomy. As a result, they would attempt to redirect the patient and convince him to stay to receive care.

What about the rest of the victims of the mass-casualty incident—the other passengers in the various cars? How do you balance a desire for justice and equal distribution of care, with beneficence, your desire to save as many people as possible? In this case, emergency providers could a use predefined support structure called the "START" triage system. This system uses simple decision points to estimate how likely it is that an individual victim of a mass casualty incident can actually benefit from your care. If a victim is unlikely to survive despite your best efforts in a setting like this with multiple wounded, your resources might best be spent elsewhere.[2]

This is a truly challenging concept to accept. It is tempting in these moments to just keep working on the individual, no matter the odds. From personal experience, I know tunnel vision can easily set in; you hyper-focus your care on one patient and may struggle to contextualize them within the broader picture. However, if your goal really is to make your actions in a crisis line up with your deepest values, then the best decision might be to move on.

Without a clearly defined ethical framework on which to base your decisions, actions in these complex situations may be inconsistent, inefficient, or subject to potential bias. With a well-developed ethical framework, you can be more certain you are making decisions that do align with your deepest values, even in high-pressure moments.

So, how do you define your moral principles? The choice is, of course, intensely personal, as it has much to do with how you view your role in the universe. You might have had an ethics module in school, or your values might be encoded in the elements of culture among a group, like the Hippocratic Oath which most medical providers take. Sometimes, professional organizations will also provide sets of guiding principles you can leverage and apply.[3]

At all times though, your actions speak the loudest about your core values. You might say you first do no harm, but do your actions during a crisis line up with these most fundamental beliefs? Just as they can complicate our ability to deploy technical skills, the pressure, uncertainty, and potential impact inherent in an emergency situation can complicate your ability to identify the "most right" way to act. Your decisions in these critical moments do more to show your guiding principles—and those of your team or organization—than any number of historical oaths you might have taken. Ultimately, responsibility to act in accordance with your principles lies squarely on your own shoulders.

Take Action

Studying ethics can sometimes be uncomfortable and challenging in a way that building other aspects of your emergency mind are not. Ethics makes you confront things like life and death, suffering, loss, and injustice in ways you might typically try to avoid. Almost by definition, the problems you deal with in this realm are sticky, complicated, and challenging. However, the time you devote to considering the deeper parts of what you believe and what type of person you want to be is time well spent.

One way to start exploring the ethics of acting during a crisis is to consider specific cases that you might be likely to face. Working through these cases in teams can be extremely helpful, as you might find unanticipated blind spots in your logic and ethical concepts that trusted teammates can help you explore. Ideally, these example cases would be handed down from more senior providers based on real-life situations they had encountered. As you work through these examples, you can draw larger lessons about the ethics you want to employ and start cross-applying them to other situations.

If a particular dilemma is likely to be encountered routinely, you and your team should think through its implications ahead of time and, whenever possible, develop consensus protocols on how to proceed. For example, adherents to the Jehovah's Witnesses faith generally do not accept transfusions of blood products. This belief could potentially create dilemmas between the principles of autonomy (electing which care to receive) and non-maleficence (not withholding life-saving care), especially if patients are unable to speak for themselves during a crisis. If you work in an organization that serves multiple practitioners of this faith, you might consider developing protocols in conjunction with members of the relevant community to help guide decision making during emergencies.

See Also

03 | Practice the Discipline of "Suboptimal"

09 | Harness the Wisdom of the Room

23 | Treat the Individual and the Field

19

FAVOR PRAXIS OVER THEORY

Acting during a crisis requires operating from the "solution space" created by the overlap of what is theoretically best practice and what is actually possible at the moment of a particular emergency. Praxis—the application of abstract knowledge to real life—is the realm of the emergency mind. Learning to identify what will actually work at the cutting edge of the crisis is a key skill in performing under pressure.

During the Apollo 13 mission to the moon in April 1970, an explosion in the oxygen tank forced the three-astronaut crew to leave their normal location in the spacecraft and rely on the lunar landing module as a "lifeboat." Unfortunately, the carbon dioxide scrubbers in the lunar module were not intended to function at the level the crew would need for very long. As a result, the astronauts' survival hinged on successfully hacking together whatever components were available to force the scrubbers to function outside their initial design parameters.

The problem, which famously involved NASA ground crews working to fit a "square peg into a round hole," was eventually solved, and thankfully all three crew members survived. Asked later about his thoughts on the solution the ground crew invented, Commander Jim Lovell said, "the contraption wasn't very handsome, but it worked."[1,2]

Given enough time and resources, the experts at NASA could certainly have developed alternate ways to remove carbon dioxide from the spacecraft—methods that were more efficient, long lasting, or had a more "handsome" design. By that point, however, the Apollo 13 astronauts might have suffocated; what the crew needed at that moment was not the theoretically best solution in a perfect world, but something that would keep them alive right then in the world they found themselves in.

Back on Earth, our needs in a crisis are very similar. While elegance is always appreciated, functionality and practicality are generally the highest design virtues in an emergency. Praxis—the application of the ideal to real life—beats theory when lives are on the line. No matter how "perfect" a solution to a problem may appear on paper, if it's impossible to implement when and where an emergency is happening, it is not the correct response.

For any given emergency, you can create a "solution space"—a Venn diagram overlap of what is theoretically best practice and what can actually be delivered in the moment. Since the edges of this solution space depend on what is possible during a particular crisis, the more informed you are about the emergent conditions and your resources, the better optimized your actions can be. Collecting, analyzing, and presenting relevant data to decision makers on the ground is therefore critically important for teams responding to an emergency.

For example, imagine you're working in a remote hospital, and you need to transport an extremely sick patient to a larger facility with more resources and specialist care. Based on your location, there are two ways to transport your patient: by ground ambulance, which would take about four hours, or by helicopter, which would take around one hour. You've done everything you can to stabilize your patient, but your hospital simply does not have the right tools to deliver the care she desperately needs. Speed of transport is your top priority, so the best solution on paper is flying her via helicopter. However if high winds and rough flying conditions prevent the helicopter crew from landing safely on a particular day, then helicopter transport is not in your solution space at that time.[3]

Which data are "relevant" to determining a solution space? It depends on the specific situation. For example, at this rural hospital, data on wind patterns and the availability of helicopter transport would obviously be important. For a tactical response team working in a hostile area, intelligence on the potential positions and capabilities of the opposing forces might be the most crucial. Generally speaking, the individuals responsible for making decisions on the front line of the emergency will be the most capable of identifying which information is most needed to determine the solution space.[4]

Finding the optimal strategy during an emergency is about balancing the tension between the on-paper best solution and the costs (time and resources) of executing that solution. So, making critical decisions well requires understanding the relative importance of "correctness" versus cost for that specific situation in that moment. Stable or slow-burning situations with well-resourced teams might benefit from the thoughtful application of more theoretically correct solutions. Unstable situations in which conditions are rapidly changing might be better served by less ideal solutions that can be implemented more quickly and with lower resource cost.

As an example, consider how to "best" dose the antibiotic vancomycin for a particular patient in the emergency department. When used intravenously to treat bacterial infections, the typical initial dose of vancomycin for a patient with normally functioning kidneys is 15-20mg/kg. If your patient weighs 70kg, the appropriate first dose would be 1050-1400mg of vancomycin.

During my residency training, several of the emergency departments I worked in would routinely stock ready-made 1g bags of vancomycin in patient care areas, but required pharmacists to mix other doses on an on-demand basis. Consequently, I could start delivering 1000mg of vancomycin within a few moments, while delivering the more technically correct 1050mg would have required the pharmacy to specially mix a different dose and transport it to the emergency department.[5]

In the case of a patient fighting an overwhelming bacterial infection, initiating early antibiotic therapy is crucially important, and you could expect the efficacy of 1000mg vs 1050mg of vancomycin for most adult patients to be quite similar. Given these facts and the probable time delay between being able to administer the two doses, the best option here is likely not the most technically correct (1050mg), but the dose you can actually accomplish now (1000mg).

Importantly, as the environment in which an emergency takes place changes, so too does the set of practical and optimal actions; performing during a crisis involves dynamically adapting to changing environmental circumstances. Understanding how to make trade-offs between theoretical precision and practicality requires a deep knowledge not only of how your craft is supposed to function, but also of the details of your environment and the resources at your disposal at this exact time. If, for example, your hospital changes their stocking practice to regularly carry premixed 1.25g bags of vancomycin in patient-care areas, the best option for your 70kg patient would also change.

At the systems and organizational level, designing for effective emergency care requires developing protocols that reflect the realities of optimizing for praxis over theory. These protocols must also be flexible enough to adapt when realities change. Institutional policies that take hard-line theoretical approaches—for example requiring that all patients receive exactly 15mg/kg of vancomycin, or that all critically-ill patients be transported by helicopter, not ground ambulance—set the stage for delay or failure as practitioners face unnecessary tension trying to adapt approaches both to exigent reality and overarching policy. Conversely, protocols developed with guidance from crews who are regularly "in the dirt" have the best chance of balancing theoretical best practices and operational knowledge to support efficient and flexible emergency responses.

As an important final note, acknowledging the realities of the situation and operating within your solution space does not mean that you resign yourself to never improving a situation, or that you accept suboptimal solutions. Identifying gaps between how you can perform at the moment and how you would want to perform in theory is an important first step in redesigning systems, inventing new strategies and tools, and advocating for broader change.

Take Action

One of the most important points of the vancomycin dosing story is how easy it would be to not know what dose of medication was stocked where, or even that different preparations were stocked in different places. At the time, there were no signs posted indicating which medications were stocked in which location. The issue was only discovered when some curious individuals started investigating delays in antibiotic dosing.

One of the best ways you can start to consider the details of praxis and theory in your field is to explore deeply the actual mechanisms that must function correctly for you to deliver your skill. Get curious about how the sausage is made, so to speak. Lean into learning both deeply in your chosen skills, and laterally into the adjacent skills that help you and your team succeed.

Ask people in different parts of your team how they function, and what barriers they face. Chances are high you will find some version of the vancomycin stocking problem that you were not previously aware of. When you do, run mental simulations of your normal workflow to see where you might improve your response with your new, more practical knowledge.

As a junior, you might also ask more senior operators what "textbook" answers—like exactly dosing vancomycin at 15mg/kg—they no longer use in the field, and how they came to change their approach. If a situation is particularly tense and discussion is not an option, you can always imagine the response you would choose and observe more senior operators to see if their behavior aligns with your imagined response. When you find differences, try to work backward to figure out why and how they arrived at these choices. Did they have a case that showed an exception to a rule? Do they know something different about how vancomycin is stocked?

Baseball legend Yogi Berra famously said, "In theory there is no difference between theory and practice. In practice, there is." Since practice is where you'll be responding to emergencies, digging into that difference is critical.

See Also

06 | Practice *Wabi-Sabi*
13 | Eliminate Unnecessary Opportunities for Failure
20 | Rapidly Accept Reality

20

RAPIDLY ACCEPT REALITY

The faster you're able to process and accept the reality of a situation, the better you'll be able to perform. Energy spent denying, complaining, or wishing things were different is energy you cannot use to respond to a crisis. You must be vigilant to recognize when a situation has changed and adapt to it. Importantly, rapidly accepting reality does NOT mean that you accept or agree with what is happening, just that you adapt to it in order to do your best work.

During the battle of Thermopylae in 480 BCE, an alliance of Greek soldiers defended their homes against an overwhelmingly larger Persian force. At one point, the arrows of the Persian army were said to be so numerous that they would block out the sun. Hearing this report, a Spartan warrior named Dienekes is said to have responded "*In umbra igitur pugnabimus,*" which translates roughly as, "Well then, won't it be nice to fight in the shade?"[1]

Dienekes' response holds a critical lesson for building your emergency mind. You don't choose the details of the emergencies that come your way—where or when they happen, or the type of challenges they bring. You certainly don't choose the number of arrows an opposing army sends your way. What you do choose, however, is how you adapt to, and accept, the situation.

From the first moments of an emergency, you choose whether you run away or stand and fight in the shade. Depending on the type of crisis you're facing, this might be a literal, physical choice—such as that faced by law enforcement officers or members of the military when confronted by direct physical threats—or a more metaphorical, mental choice. The first and most important aspect of choosing to stand and deliver is to rapidly accept the situation you and your team are facing.

Accepting reality allows you to concentrate more of your energy on solving the problem at hand. Screaming, lamenting, or wishing the situation were different will not change it, any more than Dienekes could have stopped the arrows by wishing they were not there. The energy you spend on denial, avoidance, or complaining is energy you cannot use to apply your craft.

For example, when you attempt to place a breathing tube in a critically ill patient in the emergency department, your initial attempt may falter. If so, you will need to change tactics and try something else. The more rapidly you're able to accept that the initial technique isn't working, the quicker and more smoothly you can pivot to your backup plan. Conversely, if you refuse to change approaches and acknowledge the difficulty you're having, you could end up making repeated failed attempts with that same technique, and your patient will likely suffer as a result. Data from studies on emergency airway management repeatedly show that an important factor in cases with bad outcomes is the reticence of the provider to acknowledge that the intubation is failing and that rescue techniques are needed.[2]

From an outside perspective, starting to work with what you have is clearly the superior choice to wasting energy wishing things were different. The more efficiently you can pivot to align yourself with the new reality, the more effective your emergency response will be. Logistically though, rapid acceptance and pivoting can be difficult to accomplish, either because you don't recognize that you need to accept a new situation, or because you don't want to accept it.

Recognizing a volley of arrows flying at you is relatively easy compared to catching the often much more subtle clues that suggest the ground is shifting beneath you during a crisis. Without active effort to consistently compare your mental model of the situation with the ground truth of the world around you, it's easy to miss the need to adapt and pivot. Author Laurence Gonzales, in his book *Deep Survival* on the mindset of individuals and groups in extreme accidents and survival events, put it this way, "In an environment that has high objective hazards, the longer it takes to dislodge the imagined world in favor of the real one, the greater the risk."[3]

For example, imagine a team of paramedics transporting a patient experiencing an acute flare of chronic obstructive pulmonary disease (COPD). Following their initial assessment, they activate their treatment protocols and place the patient on inhaled medications and non-invasive breathing support. A few minutes, later, when the patient is not improving, they turn up the rates and re-dose the medication. A few minutes after that, the cycle repeats itself with more COPD treatment. As they hit the gas and rush to the hospital, they likely start to get the sense they were missing something. Why, they might ask, was their patient getting worse when they were delivering all the "right" treatments?

They were, in fact, delivering appropriate COPD care—but had failed to recognize that the non-invasive breathing support had led to the patient suffering a ruptured lung—a potential complication that would not respond to COPD treatments. In this case, they had fixed their minds on the initial model of reality and had failed to dislodge their imagined world in favor of the real one.[4]

The greater your cognitive overload during a crisis and the greater the number of input streams requiring your attention, the more likely you are to miss, or subconsciously ignore, subtle cues to change direction. Confirmation bias—the mind's tendency to overweigh data that support a current hypothesis and discount data that refute it—also plays a significant role and may keep you "locked in" to a particular mental model, making it more challenging to acknowledge an important situational change.

Another reason you might not succeed at rapidly accepting a new reality is that you just don't want to. Often times, the situations you face when responding to emergencies are outrageously rough. They can be mentally, physically, or emotionally draining, and often are all three. Sometimes the situations are so extreme that they threaten to overwhelm you; not accepting the reality you see can feel psychologically safer than adapting to it. No matter how hard the situation is though, responding effectively requires that you move past this, that you stand up to the arrows of what is happening and fight in the shade.

In these cases, it is crucial to remember that rapidly accepting the reality of a situation does not mean that you approve of or like what is happening. This is especially helpful when the situation you face is profoundly emotionally charged or viscerally disturbing—for example, an emergency medical team working on a severely burned child whose injuries are the result of neglect. You do *not* condone what happened, you are *not* okay with it, but you *will* accept it and move forward because that child needs you. Energy you spend at the beginning of the case being angry and lamenting what happened is energy you cannot use to help the child.

Additionally, generating an emotionally even response at the beginning of a case does not mean you do not feel or need to process emotions. You do. We all do. It simply means that you work to devote as much of your resources as possible to the people who need you when their need is greatest. At the end of a shift or during a break in the action, reflecting on the emotions and thoughts that arise with difficult emergency responses is crucial. This is an important part of processing what happened and growing as individuals and as a team.

As a final note, it is worth thinking about the wry grin that must have accompanied Dienekes' pithy reply. Personally, when I face the arrows of uncertain and challenging circumstances—when I am trying hard to accept the reality of a difficult situation—channeling Dienekes' dark humor helps me recommit to fighting in the shade. As the Stoic philosopher and Roman emperor Marcus Aurelius is reported to have said, "Death smiles at us all; all we can do is smile back."

Take Action

When performing under pressure, you must always be vigilant and proactive, continually asking yourself if the situation you are addressing has changed. Are there new arrows heading your way? Actively seeking disconfirming evidence—asking yourself and others what you are missing that could lead to a different conclusion—is one way to overcome confirmation bias and increase the chances of recognizing a shift in circumstances. As Gonzales says, again about survivors of serious accidents, "To the survivor's mind, all cues are important. They carry information. So, a survivor expects the world to keep changing and keeps his senses always tuned to: What's up? The survivor is continuously adapting."[3]

Continuing our example with the paramedic team, when the patient failed to respond to the initial treatment, the paramedics might have said to each other some version of, "Okay, our hypothesis is COPD, but our patient is not improving. What are we missing? How do we need to adapt our mental model?" In your personal practice, try different versions of similar statements that vocalize your current hypothesis and ask for different ideas. Find one that feels natural and then put it to work.

You can address the other side of the coin—not wanting to accept reality—by practicing the acceptance of small inconveniences or minor difficult events. When you face some small situation, like spilling your coffee or lightly twisting your ankle, see how rapidly you can adapt and accept the new circumstance. Try saying out loud some version of, "Okay, this is what's happening now." Or, "This is suboptimal," as described in Chapter 3, Practice the Discipline of "Suboptimal." When you find a technique that seems to work, gradually ramp up the pressure and try it in more and more serious circumstances. When all else fails, remember Dienekes and the arrows, and try to enjoy the shade.

See Also

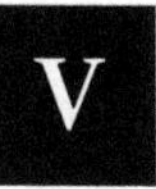

BALANCING
COMPETING FORCES

21

SEE THE FOREST AND THE LEAF

Optimizing your performance during emergencies requires balancing attention between a tight focus on individual details (the leaves) and a broad focus on the whole field (the forest). Some circumstances will require your focus to be either completely tight or completely broad. As an intelligent default, your attention should be skewed toward zoomed-in, but not completely. When you tell your teammates where your focus is directed and why, they can better understand your priorities and efficiently coordinate efforts.

Your patient just took a turn for the worse, and his blood pressure is dropping rapidly as the infection he is fighting threatens to overwhelm him. Despite your treatments, he is not getting better, so you decide to place a central line into the internal jugular vein in his neck to deliver more medications.

Fast forward a few minutes and you are midway through the procedure. Wearing a full kit of sterile gear with your patient under a plastic sheet, you are attempting to slide one end of an approximately 1.4mm-diameter guidewire into the 3mm opening of a dilator. Your gloves are slick with blood from the initial steps, which happened to be more challenging than you'd expected. Your patient, confused from his low blood pressure, keeps moving his head and accidentally pulling at the wire. You take a deep breath and concentrate more intently, your vision narrowing to a tight focus as you continue trying to get the wire into place.

Just as you are about to about to succeed, a teammate rushes into the room and pulls your attention toward a new crisis—a serious accident occurred nearby, and two badly injured people are arriving momentarily. Out of the twenty or so patients currently in the department, which two can you most safely move out of their rooms to clear space? Which resources should you activate to balance the needs of these incoming victims with the resources your other patients already require? Is that guidewire in place yet?

While many branches of medicine are set up to see patients individually in series, emergencies require you to potentially divide your attention across changing numbers of patients whom you see in parallel. This structure can force you to make complex decisions about resource allocation while simultaneously remaining focused on the highly technical details of a procedure like this central-line placement. So, how do you effectively balance attention and mental energy between a broad view of everything (the whole forest) and a hyper-focused view of a single thing (one leaf on one tree) during a crisis?

If your field of view is too broad, your attention can scatter, and performance on individual, mission-critical tasks might falter as a result. Conversely, if your field of view is too narrow, you could miss crucial events happening elsewhere, or fail to prioritize scarce resources as actions are performed without a broader context. The goal is to balance the tension between seeing the whole forest and examining the single leaf so you can flexibly deep-focus your attention as needed while still remaining responsive to the broader situation.

Unsurprisingly, balanced focus like this is not developed without concentrated effort. Determining the proper depth of focus you need to hold at a particular point during an emergency involves setting an intelligent default, proactively identifying situations that require one extreme of focus, and being flexible enough to dynamically transition as situations change.

During routine operations in the high-stakes environment of an emergency department, the best default is typically skewed somewhat more toward "zoomed in" than "zoomed out." You generally want the majority of your focus to be on the patient in front of you, with some attention devoted to scanning for threats or critical signals throughout the rest of your department. Importantly, this also allows you to pivot quickly if a sicker patient arrives unexpectedly or help is rapidly needed elsewhere.

In some circumstances—like performing a complicated central-line placement, inserting a chest tube, or performing a spinal tap—the entirety of your focus needs to be on the task at hand, with little if any attention given to the rest of the department's operations. In these "heads down" moments, other responsibilities or tasks—even important ones—can distract you and lead to errors. Consequently, those other responsibilities must be avoided or offloaded.

A useful model of this type of focus comes from the airline industry which mandates that when a plane is below 10,000 feet—a critical phase of flight during takeoff or landing—only the actions required to safely fly the plane and conversation about those actions are permitted.[1,2] Sometimes called the "Sterile Cockpit Rule," this process helps flight crews and their support teams eliminate potential sources of error or distraction during the most focus-intensive phases of their operations.

By discussing the concept of the sterile cockpit with your team ahead of time, you can help individuals shift focus during particularly critical moments in an emergency response. Logistically, this could be accomplished by having default protocols like a mandated "sterile cockpit" during an intubation between the time the anesthetic medications have been administered and the time the breathing tube is secure. Alternatively, you could train a trigger phrase such as, "Okay, team. Sterile cockpit now," to alert team members to important changes in focus goals.[3] Proactively discussing the need for this type of hyper-focus can help alleviate potential friction when some team member's concerns or non-essential issues must be deferred.

Unlike in the airline industry, where pilots only fly one plane at a time, emergency medical providers often find themselves handling multiple sick patients simultaneously. In these circumstances, it might not be possible, or even desirable, to completely restrict your focus to a single patient. Here, communication and delegation are key, and cognitively offloading some of your thinking to skilled team members helps you deploy your focus where you need it the most. For example, consider how you would manage placing a central line in one patient while another patient in a different room had a critically low blood pressure. Focusing on the line placement is crucial, but losing sight of the second patient could be dangerous.

In this (very common) situation, you might start by explaining this tension to your team, and then ask one team member to check on the other patient frequently. Instruct that person to interrupt your line placement for orders if the blood pressure drops below a certain threshold. Again, clear communication about where your focus will be and why is crucial to optimize team efforts in this type of scenario.

Immediately after a "zoom in" situation—right after the central line has been successfully placed for example—is a key time to consciously perform a "zoomed out" analysis of your department. Since your attention has been focused in one room for so long, much might have changed elsewhere; recompiling your mental model of your department is crucial to make sure it still accurately captures the reality of what you are facing.

You could recover your sense of the department by briefly looking through each individual patient chart. However, it is usually more effective to "take the pulse" of the department with whatever high-level team member has been managing the department while you were heads down. As you do this, make sure you develop an understanding of the department as a whole without getting bogged down in the details of any one patient. When all the needs are understood, you'll be able to determine the best order of next operations, and the team can swing back to a default depth of focus.

As the situations you and your team respond to change and evolve, so too does your optimal balance of breadth vs depth of focus. The ability to consciously and dynamically change focus is an important skill—and one you will use over and over again in responding to emergencies.

Take Action

In the emergency department, you can practice leaf-to-forest transitions by challenging yourself to always be able to name the department's sickest patient at any given time. It might not be the patient you're working on, and in a large department, it might not even be one of your patients at all. Asking yourself this question forces you to periodically evaluate the needs of the whole department and practice zooming out and then zooming back in.

Sometimes recompiling your mental model of the department can be done in a structured, formal way. For example, I worked in one emergency department where the leadership team was expected to meet briefly every two hours to "run the board" and identify potential challenges. Other times it can be done more informally where you challenge yourself proactively to lift your head up periodically and get a sense of the field. Improving your passive awareness in this way of what other operators are doing will always be helpful.

Conversely, a good initial exercise to develop forest-to-leaf transitions is to pick out the contributions of specific instruments while listening to music. You can start by listening to a song you know well and try to transition your attention sequentially between individual instruments. For example, you might focus first on the bass guitar, then the backup vocals, then the lead guitar, etc. When that becomes too easy, practice transitioning your attention back and forth between a broad focus incorporating the whole song and a tight focus on one particular instrument.[4]

See Also

22

FIND YOUR LOCUS OF CONTROL

Clearly identifying what you do and do not control helps you focus your resources and attention where they can make the most difference. Energy spent chasing things you do not control is energy you cannot bring to bear on a crisis. Ask yourself what you can accomplish right now to make this situation better with what you have. Concentrating on this question before, during, and after a crisis will help you eliminate performance anxiety, recognize where you can make the greatest difference, and clarify where you should focus your future training.

The Stoic philosopher Epictetus said, "Things in our control are opinion, pursuit, desire, aversion, and, in a word, whatever are our own actions. Things not in our control are body, property, reputation, command, and, in one word, whatever are not our own actions."[1] Put another way, there are two types of things in the universe—the relatively small set of things over which you have control, and the much, much larger set of things you do not control.

During an emergency you control your actions, the vast majority of your thoughts, many of your responses to stimuli, and your sense of mission and purpose. You do not control when an emergency happens, the details of the crisis you face, the actions of anyone else involved, or essentially anything else.

Most importantly, you do not control the outcome of the crisis. You only your performance before, during, and after. Like an archer, you may practice diligently and take skillful aim at the target, but once the arrow leaves your bow it is no longer under your control.

With a finite amount of attention and energy to deploy, identifying the limits of what you control—finding your sphere of influence—is crucial to improving your performance. For example, if you're the victim of a hit-and-run accident on a highway, focusing on the other driver's criminal behavior draws your attention away from safely getting yourself and your family out of the middle of the road. While you might be justifiably angry at the other driver, those thoughts and feelings are not a helpful use of your attention at that moment. With this sphere of influence in mind, one of the most powerful questions you can ask during an emergency is "what can I (or my team) do right now to make this situation better?"[2]

Asking this question builds a Venn diagram between what the patient or situation needs and where you have the ability to act. With subtle changes, this question can be useful before a crisis to facilitate preparation for whatever is incoming, during a crisis to help you focus on taking efficient and skilled action, and after a crisis to aid in identifying reusable lessons for further training.

Before the start of an emergency, you can ask what you and your team are capable of doing right now to improve your readiness to perform under pressure. If you're expecting a specific type of crisis, asking this question can help you cut through any preperformance anxiety you might be feeling and refocus your mind where it can be of use. For example, imagine you're alerted to an incoming pediatric patient suffering a severe asthma attack. Airway management for young children can be extremely complicated and anxiety-provoking, even for experienced providers. Identifying your locus of control encourages you to shift away from anxious thoughts to what you and your team can do to prepared. You cannot control the child's illness, but you do control your actions and can use your time to set up equipment and review proper dosing of medications.

During a crisis, asking where you have control can keep you focused on moving forward despite setbacks or challenging circumstances. Imagine you're a pilot working to land a plane after a catastrophic engine failure. It might be tempting to concentrate on the broken engine, blame the mechanics, or wish the wind patterns were different. Instead, asking what you do control helps focus your energy on doing everything possible to land the plane safely with the remaining engines.

As an emergency progresses, your locus of control will likely change. Each time there is a new evolution in the problem you face, ask yourself what you can do right now to make the situation better—either formally as a group or internally to yourself. That continued questioning will keep you pointed in the right direction.

After the crisis has resolved, understanding where you had control and where you did not is crucial to evaluate how you performed and identify areas for improvement. To grow after a crisis, you need to distinguish between your performance—how you succeeded in the domains in which you had control—and the outcome, which is never totally under your control. Returning to the metaphor of the archer, performance is how you aimed the shot, drew back the bow, and loosed the arrow, while outcome is what happened after the arrow left your bow, including whether or not it hit the target.

Successfully parsing the details of what happened into performance and outcome in order to facilitate more accurate learning is termed "fielding" by decision-making expert and former poker champion Annie Duke.[3] Certainly, the outcome of a case informs your judgment of your performance—hitting the target is absolutely important—but failing to distinguish where you had control and where you did not can seriously hamper your ability to improve.

Imagine, for example a serious trauma in which a young woman was struck by a car and sustained a fractured pelvis. You quickly identified the injury and placed a pelvic binder device, but she had suffered serious internal bleeding en route from the scene and died shortly after arriving in your emergency department.

How would you field this case? If you were entirely outcome-focused, you might fixate on your patient's death—clearly a difficult and sad outcome. As a result, you might lose confidence in your ability to treat patients, or inappropriately berate your team, either of which could compromise your actions during the next trauma.

Conversely, a more effective version of fielding would dissect out where you had control (your actions) from where you did not (whether the patient lives or dies). In this way, you could identify those areas where you could study and possibly improve your performance, regardless of the outcome.

As you seek to better focus your attention where you do have control, you will find that while you rarely can fix *everything*, you almost always can do *something* to improve yourself and your teams. When you find it, do it.

Take Action

The best way to practice finding your locus of control is to jump in and ask what you can do right now to make a situation better. If that question feels too difficult or complex, start by looking for three things that you control during a situation. If three is too many, start by identifying one single thing that you control during a crisis.

When you first begin training your emergency mind, it can feel like absolutely nothing is within your control. In this case, a good place to start is with the breath. You almost always have control over your own breath. Just take a deep inhale and a deep exhale, and then ask yourself again where you have control. It's deceptively simple, and taking a single deep breath like this can be a useful reset that will often help you think more clearly about where you have the ability to make a difference. As you keep training, practice noticing your breathing during tense situations, and consciously exert control to slow down and improve your oxygenation.[4]

After an emergency has passed, practice recognizing that the outcome of the situation is not the same as your performance. Review what happened and ask yourself where you had control and what was outside your power. Being deeply honest during this process can help you answer two questions: Do I take on burdens that I might not need to? Where can I improve my skills?

See Also

23

TREAT THE INDIVIDUAL AND THE FIELD

Since emergencies often require deploying scarce resources across multiple patients with different needs, caring for an individual must be done within the broader context of the overall mission. Sometimes, this means the needs of an individual must be subjugated to the needs of the set of patients you are treating. Having an up-to-date mental model of the whole field is necessary to navigate this tension. Protocols like triage and code-blue responses can be used to rebalance resources as needs change.

As an emergency medical provider, your two goals are to take care of the patients who are already in your emergency department, and to maintain reserve capacity to treat additional individuals who might need you later. When I was auditioning for a spot in emergency residency training, Erik Antonsen, MD PhD, then one of the senior residents, explained it this way:

See this guy in front of you with the minor chest pain? Behind him, in the waiting room, are five other people with chest pain who are waiting to be seen. We don't know if they're low risk or not yet since we haven't seen them. Behind those folks are some number of other people with chest pain in ambulances on their way in. And behind them are folks at home thinking about calling 911 for their chest pain. Your job is not just to take care of this one guy. Your job is to do the best you can to take care of him in the context of the entire cone of people spreading out behind him. Those people—the ones you can't see yet—they're your patients too. Never forget that.[1]

So, how do you balance the tension between these two goals? How do you design efficient responses that incorporate both the requirements of the person in front of you and the unknown needs of potential future emergencies that might occur later? Striking this balance requires intelligently making trade-offs in resource allocation and high degrees of clarity on the specific goals and scope of your mission when you respond to a crisis.

In the emergency department, this often means you do not optimize your actions for any one single patient; you optimize your actions across the field of patients you are treating. Since that set of patients might change suddenly in the event of a disaster like a bus crash or a house fire, optimizing for the field involves maintaining spare capacity that can be rapidly spun up as needed.

For example, consider the extremely common problem of prioritizing access to a scarce resource such as a CT scanner. Each patient in the queue waiting for a CT scan is individually best served by being imaged immediately; optimizing care for an individual patient means placing them at the top of the list now, regardless of the needs of any other patients.

Within the broader context of your responsibility however, there frequently will be significant variability in the relative urgencies of individuals being imaged. Some patients—like a person seemingly experiencing an acute stroke—do need to be scanned immediately. Others—such as a patient with abdominal pain, stable vitals, and a reassuring physical exam—while no less "deserving" of those resources, would receive nearly equal benefit from being scanned now as in an hour from now. Optimizing care across the field in this context would involve prioritizing CT scans for those patients who would receive outsized benefits from immediate imaging, even if this makes some other patients wait longer.

The first step in actually accomplishing this type of optimization is to understand the environment and context in which you are responding to emergencies. For example, teams delivering care in the aftermath of a hurricane need accurate mental models of the scope of the disaster and the potential number and location of injured individuals, as well as the details of what resources they have available to meet those needs. These mental models must be flexible since the set of injured individuals, the needs of each individual, and the resources of the response team may change rapidly and often without warning.

Importantly, your decisions about assigning priorities across a group of patients will depend on your particular view of that group of patients. Individuals with different understandings of what is needed may come to different conclusions on what the most important actions are at a given moment. A pediatrician, for example, might focus primarily on the children needing emergency care and therefore prioritize delivery of care to minors at the expense of everyone else.

On one extreme end of this spectrum is the individual patient; this person cannot see the whole field, and might easily become frustrated or upset if their care seems delayed or if other patients seem to be cared for more quickly. Aiding patients in viewing their needs in a broader context might help individuals look past themselves, find deeper levels of calm, and understand the larger picture. ("I really want you to get this CT scan as soon as possible, but right now I need the scanner for a grandmother who might be having a stroke.") Helping them manage their pain and discomfort and providing additional resources, like blankets or a phone to call loved ones, can go a long way in facilitating this change of perspective.

At the systems level, balancing care for individuals and the field as a whole involves designing protocols that ensure timely access to scarce resources for those who need them most. These protocols should help focus your attention where it is most useful and aid you in maintaining flexible capacity for changes in the scope of the crisis.

Two key systems-level protocols we use in the emergency department are the triage system and the code-blue alert. Both of these protocols have extensive applications in the broader context of providing services in parallel to large groups outside the emergency department, including during other types of crises and in times of routine operation. In a sense, they are opposites; triage is used to effectively distribute resources across a wide area, while a code blue is used to rapidly concentrate them at a single point.

During the triage process, individual patients are sorted on arrival to the emergency department in an effort to properly match them with the level of resources they need. For the neediest cases, this means rapidly devoting resources to their treatment. For more stable patients, this could mean waiting extended periods to receive attention and care.

Triaging helps your system maintain an up-to-date mental model of the group's needs and facilitates rapidly changing the distribution of resources to match these needs. Without a triage process, individuals might be treated in the order of their arrival or based on social privilege of some form, likely resulting in suboptimal delivery of care.

Code-blue alerts are activated when a patient suffers a cardiac arrest, which requires a significant concentration of resources for effective treatment. Personnel and specialized equipment and medication must be delivered to the patient's location and activated immediately, typically regardless of other on-going needs elsewhere in the hospital. Activating a code blue—or other similar team activations, like trauma team activations, obstetric team activations, etc.—alerts providers that the field has changed significantly and abruptly. The old mental models of workflow need to be abandoned and rapidly replaced by new ones.[2]

Where types of protocols like triage or codes exist, you need to study how they work and train on how to best use them. Where they don't, you need to proactively think about what types of decision-support structures could help you hold an accurate and flexible model of the field, and keep evolving that model as the nature of the emergency changes. Above all, you need to remember the whole scope of your mission, not just the obvious parts directly in front of you. As Dr. Antonsen said, "Those people—the ones you can't see yet—they're your patients too. Never forget that."

Take Action

In any crisis, the more complete, flexible, and intelligent your mental model of the whole field is, the more effectively you can respond. Consequently, you need to actively seek out ways to contextualize your individual actions within the broader scope of your mission, and update your priorities as the situations you face continue to change.

A first step in building this skill is to pause at set intervals to actively scan the field and practice identifying the sickest individuals or those who need the most resources. Try this out on your next shift by setting a timer. Every hour (or whatever interval you like), perform a mental scan of the field and update your mental model. A more advanced method takes advantage of identifying pauses in the action to perform these scans during natural breaks in your emergency response.[3]

Where your team uses protocols like the triage system to balance individual and field needs, study how that system functions in real-life situations. Volunteer to spend time shadowing the triage providers to learn how they decide who needs what. Talk to the individuals who run code-blue responses about their thinking before, during, and after an acute event. Pay special attention to their habits immediately after returning from a code event, when they have to transition their focus from the individual back to the field. How do they accomplish this? How could you put their tools into practice and improve on them?

See Also

15 | Find the Rate-Limiting Step
18 | Start From First Principles
19 | Favor Praxis Over Theory

24

COMBINE ACTION AND ANALYSIS

Your emergency mind includes a "fast gear" that prioritizes immediate action in the face of uncertainty and a "slow gear" that prioritizes deep investigation and thoughtful experimentation. Knowing when you are forced to act immediately and when you have time to step back and analyze a situation comes with experience and training. At more junior levels, you should prioritize action first and analysis second during a crisis.

To perform successfully under pressure during an emergency, you need to develop two distinct modes of behavior. The first mode is fast, action-focused, and devoted to addressing a particular situation. It makes use of whatever knowledge and tools are available at the moment and generally seeks to address a specific goal, like helping a choking patient breathe. The second mode is more careful and exploratory. It is devoted to seeking out the best possible solution to a problem and involves gathering data, comparing options, and planning future courses of action. Generally, this second mode seeks to balance multiple different priorities such as diagnosing a patient's illness while being efficient in resource utilization.

During the response to a crisis, you must balance the strengths and weaknesses of both of these modes, and recognize which type of response is required when. Using the slower mode of action when a faster response is required is a critical mistake that can easily result in failure. During the moments you are not acting, the emergency you face can evolve rapidly, and at times irrevocably, into a more complicated and unstable situation. For example, if you found a patient in cardiac arrest and chose to slowly think through potential causes instead of starting CPR immediately, you would lose your window to act and further efforts at resuscitation would likely be futile.

Conversely, using the fast mode of action when immediate action is not needed is akin to flailing. It can be a clumsy waste of energy that could be better spent elsewhere and is likely to generate a worse solution than a more thoughtful, analytic approach. Imagine a hospital unit that activated a code-blue response team every time a patient had chest pain. Not only would this divert resources unnecessarily from areas they might otherwise be needed, it might also decrease the effectiveness of future code team activations as team members took them less seriously.

To further explore the difference between these modes, consider two patients, both presenting to an emergency department with a chief complaint of difficulty breathing and an initial oxygen saturation of 94 percent on room air.

Patient A arrives in respiratory distress after eating something that contains peanuts, a food to which she has a significant allergy. She is covered in hives and audibly wheezing. Patient B arrives short of breath and reports this condition has been building gradually over the past several months. He has a slight fever but otherwise stable vital signs.

Obviously, the optimal approach to providing emergency care differs significantly between these patients. Immediate intervention is required for Patient A, who appears to be suffering from a potentially life-threatening anaphylactic reaction. In this case, you are "forced to act," since not acting has a high probability of morbidity or mortality. Importantly, even if the diagnosis of allergic reaction were much less clear, you would still be forced to act for Patient A in response to her clinical instability and low blood pressure.[1]

For Patient B, a thoughtful approach focused on data gathering and investigation is more appropriate than immediate action. Because he is more stable than patient A, you are not forced to act immediately. Instead, you can devote energy to comparing multiple strategies of how you might best respond. When you are not forced to act, jumping into a response without further analysis of the emergency is sometimes a bit like throwing darts without looking at the dartboard. You might hit the board, but because you don't understand where you're aiming, you're much more likely to miss the target entirely and waste your darts.

So, how do you determine if you are "forced to act" at a given moment in an emergency response? First, you can be forced to act if life, limb, or significant loss is immediately on the line, and you believe that delay or inaction would result in catastrophic failure. For example, a patient with arterial bleeding after a trauma requires immediate action to stop the bleeding, or they will likely exsanguinate and die.[2] Similarly, a choking victim needs their airway cleared immediately or they will likely suffer a respiratory arrest.

Second, even if there is not an immediate threat, you can be forced to act if you recognize patterns that forecast future danger with high probability. Returning to Patient A, the constellation of hives and shortness of breath suggest anaphylaxis rather than a simple allergic reaction. Knowing that anaphylaxis can progress rapidly to cardiovascular collapse, you are forced to act immediately to prevent a more critical emergency from occurring.[3]

Finally, you are sometimes forced to act—or at least forced to strongly consider acting—if you have access to a particular resource that is only available or effective within a specific window of time. For example, in the treatment of acute stroke, thrombolytic drugs are generally only effective when delivered within four hours of the start of the symptoms. Two patients who present with identical neurological deficits, one ten minutes after they started, and one three hours after they started, would likely merit different approaches reflecting the time-sensitive nature of available treatments. In this scenario, asking when the patient was last seen well is therefore one of the most important initial questions.

Most commonly though, emergency situations require a mixed approach where combinations of immediate and slower actions are employed together. For example, on finding a patient unconscious and barely breathing, immediate action is required to deliver oxygen. Appropriate first steps would typically include immediately performing a head-tilt and jaw-thrust maneuver and administering supplemental oxygen.[4] If these maneuvers improved the patient's oxygenation, then you could proceed with a deeper, slower analysis to determine why the patient was breathing like this and what could be done about it. If not, further action-focused steps, potentially including placing the patient on a ventilator, might be needed.

As a final note, individuals and teams that are more experienced in responding to emergencies are typically better at understanding which mode of action is most appropriate when. More junior providers would do well to assume that immediate action is almost always needed first before backing off to perform deeper analyses. In this way, they are more likely to appropriately respond to critical situations even when they might not fully understand the details of what they face.

Take Action

Early in your training, it can be extremely difficult to recognize when to act and when to slow down and analyze. You can start exploring those differences by watching more experienced providers and noting when they shift gears. As they transition between those two modes, try to figure out what pattern they identified, or why they decided a different approach would be better. Do not stop them in the middle of the action to ask what they're thinking, especially if they are transitioning from a slow mode to a fast mode. Instead, take some notes about what happened and review them later.

If a senior provider suddenly goes from seated and thinking to up and active, you should try to figure out why. If you're not involved in anything critical at that moment, ask to go along. If they start running either toward or away from something, chances are very high that you need to be running, too.[5] Alternatively, if a senior provider transitions from action to a more contemplative gear, try to discover what reassuring pattern they noticed. Has the danger passed, or have they simply completed everything they had control over for the moment?

As you gain more experience, you will tend to naturally proceed in an "act first, analyze second" pattern. As this happens, work to explicitly do a "second sweep," in which you slow down and revisit your assumptions.[6] This can be very helpful in preventing errors and deepening your understanding of a case. Doing these slower walk-throughs out loud can give your more junior team members a chance to "ride along" and practice their transitions with you.

See Also

25

USE ALGORITHMIC AND CREATIVE THINKING

Algorithmic thinking is linear, follows predetermined paths, and can be used at a variety of skill and knowledge levels. Creative thinking is non-linear and relies on taking steps and leaps between often disparate areas of knowledge to form uniquely tailored solutions. Each form of problem solving has its strengths and weakness in different situations, and wiring your brain to perform involves leveraging both.

As you arrive to your shift in the emergency department, one of the senior nurses calls you urgently into a patient's room. A few hours earlier, the patient had presented in respiratory distress from a severe pneumonia. After trying multiple other options, your teammate had placed a breathing tube and started her on mechanical ventilation. Initially, she was improving, but now her oxygen saturation is dropping rapidly, the ventilator is firing multiple alarms, and her heart rate is spiking. Why is this happening, and what should you do about it?

A vast array of problems can happen whcn a patient is dependent on a ventilator, and in this case there's not nearly enough time for you to sort through them all exhaustively without a supporting structure to guide your thinking. Thankfully, you have an algorithm—called DOPES—to organize your search for the cause of low oxygen in a ventilated patient.[1]

The DOPES algorithm divides all potential problems into three categories: issues inside the patient, issues inside the ventilator, or issues involving the connection between the two. Guided by this algorithm, you're able to efficiently narrow down the field of potential problems and rapidly identify the likely culprit. In this case, it seems there's a physical blockage within the breathing tube that is preventing the ventilator from delivering breaths.

Now you know what the problem is, but how do you solve it? There is no algorithmic approach here to guide you, so you switch mental gears to a broader, non-linear, creative approach. You might consider options you've personally executed in similar situations, options you've seen someone else perform, a few ideas you read about once, and you might even generate one or two options that come from who knows where.[2]

You've seen a lot of blockages removed successfully by suctioning them out the breathing tube, so that's where you start. Unfortunately, that doesn't work, and your patient starts to decompensate even more rapidly. Time is running out.

In a burst of creative insight, you reverse the parameters of your solution—you won't suction the blockage up, you'll push the blockage down, deeper into the lung and out of the breathing tube. This is not an ideal solution, and there will likely be physiologic consequences for the patient later. At the moment, however, it is a viable solution that gets the blockage out of the way and keeps her alive. You execute your plan and watch her vital signs start to return to normal.

As highlighted in this example, both algorithmic and creative thinking are critically important for performing under pressure, each offering potential advantages and disadvantages in any given situation. Learning to best utilize each method—and how to use them together synergistically—is a key goal as you build your emergency mind.

Algorithms are sets of instructions designed to be executed in a particular way to solve a specific type of problem. Algorithmic thinking relies on using predefined approaches or decision-support tools to arrive at a solution or dictate the next appropriate action. This type of thinking is linear in that it proceeds stepwise along a known path. It is predetermined, as the path of analysis was laid out ahead of time. It is also general, in that the algorithm you follow during a crisis was designed not to solve your exact problem, but rather to be useful for a general class of problems that includes your current situation to a greater or lesser extent.

Algorithmic thinking is widespread in the provision of emergency care. The mental models describing the ABC approach to resuscitation, and the primary-secondary-tertiary approach to trauma are both examples of algorithmic thinking, as is the DOPES protocol described above. Outside of the emergency department, algorithmic thinking is employed by pilots addressing in-air emergencies, engineers working with a critical failure in a power plant, and bomb squad experts responding to a potential explosive device, among others.[3,4]

By comparison, creative or free-form thinking follows no predetermined rules and attempts to derive a unique, one-off solution for a specific problem. Where algorithmic thinking is linear, creative thinking is unstructured and can proceed dynamically between different options. Often, it involves small steps and close iterations of possibilities. In the example above, this could be something like continuing to attempt to suction the blockage but using a different type of suction device. Other times, free-form thinking makes large leaps in logic and reasoning to present a totally novel idea, like moving the blockage down instead of up. Where algorithmic thinking is explicit and easy to follow, creative thinking is usually implicit and can be difficult if not impossible to follow, even for the "thinker."[5]

Like algorithmic thinking, creative thinking is also widespread in emergency medicine, where a nearly limitless array of potential crises will force you to constantly adapt your plans to new and changing circumstances. The mental models described in Chapters 2, 3, and 6 of this book—Become a Student of Sangfroid, Practice the Discipline of "Suboptimal," and Practice *Wabi-Sabi*—all involve the use of some form of creative thinking to overcome unexpected obstacles.

Outside of the emergency department, free-form thinking is employed by jiu-jitsu players combining attacks in novel ways to submit a skilled opponent, entrepreneurs imagining disruptive solutions to previously intractable problems, sailors improvising solutions to equipment failures with whatever supplies happen to be on hand, and many, many others.[6]

Comparing these two types of thinking, emergency physician Dana Sajed, MD, describes algorithmic thinking to be like musical scales and chord progressions, and creative thinking to be like improvisational jazz.[7] To further understand these two modes of thinking, let's explore their performance under extreme conditions, the types of solutions they tend to generate, and the domain expertise required to wield them.

First, while both methods of thinking can successfully be utilized under pressure, algorithmic thinking is easier to deploy when you're exhausted, hungry, or cognitively overloaded; algorithms are the "tired moves" of emergency thinking as explored in Chapter 5. In fact, algorithms like the DOPES protocol are essentially designed to facilitate cognitive offloading, as Atul Gawande, MD MPH, discusses in one of the best-known works on the utility of algorithms in medicine, *The Checklist Manifesto*.[8]

Second, algorithms can only use the types of data that were known when the algorithm was developed can only generate a conclusion based on that data.[9] By comparison, creative thinking is unbounded both in its inputs and solutions. Even when it follows some core rules, like the logic underlying the art of a jazz solo, it is more likely than algorithmic thinking to arrive at unique solutions.

Third, since creative thinking often relies on generating connections between seemingly disparate points of information, the deeper your fund of knowledge, the stronger the tool can be for you. While the "fresh eyes" of a novice practitioner do often yield novel results, domain experts are at a distinct advantage when utilizing creative thinking, as they have both a deeper and a broader array of experiences to draw on. Algorithmic thinking, on the other hand, is largely indifferent to your level of expertise. As long as you're able to understand and execute the individual steps of an algorithm, your level of your training is typically not a factor in its function.

Most of your emergency responses will rely on a mix of the two modes of thinking, rather than on either of them exclusively. As the example of the blocked breathing tube demonstrates, algorithmic thinking can identify issues around which you can iterate and then diverge using creative thinking. Conversely, creative thinking can chart new paths around which algorithms can later be developed.

Take Action

If you are more junior in your training, starting to explore algorithmic thinking is easier than jumping immediately to creative thinking. Begin with a deep dive into the algorithms experienced providers rely on in their day-to-day work and in their most challenging cases. Ask the more senior operators around you what algorithms they use, and how they apply them.

Dig into the details of how these algorithms are constructed, where they function well, and where they break down. Mentally walk through the algorithms again and again before applying them in real life. Watch your teammates and see how they actually apply algorithmic thinking, not just how they say they do. What do those differences tell you about how the algorithms work?

Once you have a solid foundation of core knowledge and technique, a great way to explore creative thinking is by looking at the areas where algorithmic thinking starts to break down. In the example above, algorithmic thinking identified a particular problem that creative thinking could then try to solve. Visualize a group of similar scenarios where the problem was found at a different point in the DOPES algorithm. Starting from these problems, try using creative thinking to brainstorm potential solutions. If that is too easy, add in extra constraints like time pressure, power outages, or instrument failures.

Additionally, asking expert operators how they developed particular ideas can yield valuable and interesting insights. Make celebrating the artful blending of algorithmic and creative thinking part of your team's culture; share unique solutions widely and challenge teammates to develop more creative solutions to tough problems.

See Also

A PARTING CHALLENGE

I finish every episode of *The Emergency Mind Podcast* (www.emergencymind.com/podcast) by asking my guest(s) to issue a challenge to everyone listening. So, instead of ending this book by suggesting a reading list, I offer you this challenge: I challenge you to bring these mental models to life, to put them into practice, modify them, grow beyond them, and then teach me what you've learned. Specifically, I want you to get curious and start to experiment with whatever ideas in the book resonated with you the most. Nothing about this book is designed to gather dust on a shelf; everything is designed to be used.

You can start right now by honestly taking stock of what happens when you get into tough situations. Keep notes on how you currently perform under pressure. Look inward and reflect on what you see. Where are you or your team strongest under pressure, and where do you need to become stronger? What do you struggle with, and where do you excel?

Then, put on your "scientist hat" and start experimenting. Which ideas in this book spoke the loudest to you? Start putting them into practice when you feel stress and need to perform. Iterate, combine them, and generate new ideas and models of your own. Test hypotheses and take notes on what combinations work the best for you personally. Discuss these hybrid mental models with your friends and teammates and see what you can come up with. Run these experiments in your day-to-day life and run them mentally while visualizing how you would perform if you needed to save someone's life.

From a narrow and selfish perspective, I want you to do this because the person you try to save one day might very well be me. More broadly though, I believe deeply that the better each of us becomes at handling pressure, the better off we are collectively. When you and I both train to perform better in the face of real-life challenges—when we each build our emergency minds—the scope of how well we can perform during a crisis and where we can triumph under pressure expands massively.

So, get after it. Along the way, if you want more ideas, if you want to see what I am working on, or if you want to compare notes, head over to www.emergencymind.com. I would love to hear from you.

Good luck out there.
Dan

ACKNOWLEDGMENTS

I am incredibly thankful for the vast array of people I've been fortunate enough to spend time with as I've worked on this book.

First, I am deeply grateful to my editor, Janis Dworkis (www.janisdworkis.com), for her guidance, expertise, and support. The fact that I was able to work so closely with my mother as a professional was a bonus for me in this work and brought much needed joy into each wave of revisions. I am also deeply grateful to Bridget Hilton (www.bridgethilton.com) and Rachel Connors for their excellent work on the cover design.

To my family, Michael, Brittany, Mom and Dad, and to my friends—especially Amy, Bridget, Joe, Jon, Liz, Rachel, Richard, and Vlad—thank you for supporting me, pushing me, and believing in me. Thank you for reading all the early drafts, even the questionable ones, and for your guidance. This book is stronger because of you, and so am I.

To the people who trained me, who trained with me, and whom I am fortunate enough to work with at the Keck School of Medicine of USC, LAC+USC Medical Center, The Brigham and Women's/ Massachusetts General Hospital Harvard Affiliated Emergency Medicine Residency, Boston University School of Medicine / Boston Medical Center, Providence St. Joseph Hospital Eureka, and the Northern Navajo Medical Center, thank you for teaching me how to hold the line, and for instilling in me the desire to do better every shift.

To my students, it is a joy to work with you and watch you learn and grow. I am undoubtedly a better physician because of your hard work. Particular thanks go to the folks at the Emergency Medicine Student Interest Group at the Keck School of Medicine of USC who read an early draft and provided crucial feedback and direction.

To my patients, thank you for your faith in me and in my team. I am sorry for the suffering that brings you in front of me, but I promise I will do my best to never waste it. When it is my turn on the table, I will show up armed with the bravery and strength you have shown me.

Finally, to you, the reader. Thank you for the work you're doing to become better at performing under pressure. Keep your head up.

NOTES

What Is an Emergency?

1   The core components of an emergency as defined in this book—uncertainty, impact, and pressure—are built from personal experience and conversations with diverse groups of individuals who regularly perform under pressure. A similar definition is offered by authors Weisinger and Pawliw-Fry in their book *Performing Under Pressure: The Science of Doing Your Best When It Matters Most*, which is worth a read if you're interested in exploring how other groups define emergent situations. Weisinger, H. and Pawliw-Fry, JP. *Performing Under Pressure: The Science of Doing Your Best When It Matters Most*. (Currency, 2015).

2   Duke, A. *Thinking in Bets: Making Smarter Decisions When You Don't Have All the Facts* (Portfolio, 2018).

3   An important linked concept is the idea of extraneous cognitive load, which describes the mental energy you use in a circumstance that is unrelated to the task at hand. For example, if multiple alarms were going off loudly in a room while you were trying to place a delicate IV line, the energy you spent blocking out the alarms and concentrating on the IV would be extraneous cognitive load. A good review of cognitive load theory can be found in: Lovell, O. *Sweller's Cognitive Load Theory in Action* (John Catt Educational Ltd, 2020).

Emergency Mental Models

1   For an excellent explanation of mental models in general and a fascinating array of mental models used by individuals across a diverse set of fields and professions, I recommend the Farnam Street Blog, written by Shane Parish. This article is a good place to start: Farnam Street. "Mental Models: The Best Way to Make Intelligent Decisions (109 Models Explained)." https://fs.blog/mental-models/.

2   See for example: Delicce, AV. and Makaryus, AN., "Physiology, Frank Starling Law." StatPearls, 2021. https://www.ncbi.nlm.nih.gov/books/NBK470295/.

3   See for example the section on "The Science of Many Models" in Page, SE. *The Model Thinker: What You Need to Know to Make Data Work for You* (Basic Books, 2018).

01 | Find the Calm in the Storm

1   If you have never run a cardiac arrest or trained in ACLS, an obvious question might be: "Why stop every two minutes? Why not just keep doing CPR the whole time?" Functionally, the cardiac monitor that detects the electrical activity of the heart is not able to accurately detect this activity while chest compressions are ongoing. So we need to periodically pause compressions to see if the patient's heart has restarted and is able to function on its own. Minimizing these moments without compressions is one of the hallmarks of an effective resuscitation team.

2   The act of developing expertise in an area and transitioning decision making from conscious to automatic circuits is often referred to as "schema generation," or "chunking." The details of how expertise is actually developed in an area is outside the scope of the book, but it is truly fascinating. If you're interested in a deeper dive, I recommend the *Huberman Lab* podcast for the neuroanatomical details (www.youtube.com/c/andrewhubermanlab) and *Sweller's Cognitive Load Theory in Action* for details on the theory of how we learn and remember. Lovell, O. *Sweller's Cognitive Load Theory in Action* (John Catt Educational Ltd, 2020).

3   For deeper discussions of these examples—and a variety of other tools individuals and teams can use to increase efficiency during emergencies and build space to think—see the section on "Pressure

Control" in Hearns, S. *Peak Performance Under Pressure* (Class Professional Publishing, 2019).

4   The original quote reads "For in the same degree in which a man's mind is nearer to freedom from all passion, in the same degree also is it nearer to strength." Aurelius, M. *Meditations.* Long, G. (Trans). http://classics.mit.edu/Antoninus/meditations.html.

02 | Become a Student of Sangfroid

1   James Clear's book *Atomic Habits* has a great deal to say about this idea. See for example, the section on "How to Stop Procrastinating by Using the Two-Minute Rule." Clear, J. *Atomic Habits: An Easy & Proven Way to Build Good Habits & Break Bad Ones* (Avery, 2018).

2   It's worth pressing on this point a bit, especially since it is easy when we start training to focus only on the gap between ourselves and individuals who are already established experts in sangfroid. The goal is to make small improvements under pressure, not to attain perfection. If you are practicing sangfroid and you are one percent better than you were on your previous shift, you're on the right path. For more about the importance of focusing on process and improvement over an end goal, consider reading: Le Cunff, A. "The Nirvana Fallacy: when perfectionism leads to unrealistic solutions." *Ness Labs.* https://nesslabs.com/nirvana-fallacy.

03 | Practice the Discipline of "Suboptimal"

1   In this section, because we are focusing on the response and not the error, I gloss over the differences between "mistakes" and "slips, trips, or lapses," which technically are different categories of errors. That said, if you're interested in a deeper dive into error, consider the section on "Human Error" in Rutherford, G (Ed). *Human Factors in Paramedic Practice* (Class Professional Publishing, 2020).

2   As an alternative example, a teammate of mine uses the phrase, "Uh-oh SpaghettiOs™," which he borrowed from a decades-old television commercial.

3   The Harvard T.H. Chan School of Public Health offers a great introduction to root cause analyses in a YouTube video called "How To Conduct a Root Cause Analysis of a Critical Incident." https://www.youtube.com/watch?v=iIis4YloV8Q&t=121s.

04 | Apply Graduated Pressure

1   A video explaining the central line insertion training process using a simulator can be found at the New York City Health and Hospitals Simulation Center website, https://www.nychealthandhospitals.org/simulationcenter/central-line-placement-skills/.

2   The neuroscience of how our brains process failures and modulate neuroplasticity to adjust and learn is fascinating but outside the scope of this book. If you're interested in a deeper dive in understanding the science of why failures are important for learning, I recommend starting with this episode of the *Huberman Labs* podcast: Huberman, A. (host). "How to Learn Faster by Using Failures, Movement & Balance." *Huberman Labs*. Episode 7. https://podcasts.apple.com/ca/podcast/how-to-learn-faster-by-using-failures-movement-balance/id1545953110?i=1000509076366.

3   Clear, J. "The Goldilocks Rule: How to Stay Motivated in Life and Business." www.JamesClear.com/Goldilocks-Rule.

05 | Train Your Tired Moves

1   Salgado, R. Personal communication, 2019.

2   While delivering breaths to a patient via a BVM is one of the first skills taught in airway management, it is not simple. Overtraining BVM until it becomes a tired move is critical for emergency providers. See for example, this article from the *Journal of Emergency Medical Services* which reviews the basics of BVM use. Rock, M. "The Dos and Don'ts of Bag-Valve Mask Ventilation," JEMS, 2014. https://www.jems.com/patient-care/dos-and-don-ts-bag-valve-mask-ventilatio/.

3   For an excellent description of performing premortem evaluations by one of the known thought leaders in decision making under real-life conditions, consider this article in the *Harvard Business Review* by Gary Klein: Klein, G. "Performing a Project Premortem," *Harvard Business Review*, 2007. https://hbr.org/2007/09/performing-a-project-premortem.

4   See for example the US National Transportation Safety Board's rich data on accidents in the airline industry. https://www.ntsb.gov/investigations/AccidentReports/Pages/aviation.aspx.

06 | Practice *Wabi-Sabi*

1   If you're interested in a deeper dive into the details of the philosophy and applications of *wabi-sabi*, I suggest *Wabi-Sabi for Artists, Designers, Poets & Philosophers*, by Leonard Koren. It is an excellent, easily accessible book. Koren, L. *Wabi-Sabi for Artists, Designers, Poets & Philosophers* (Stone Bridge Press, 1994).

2   The distinctions between these concepts are artificial, and attempting to subdivide and incrementally approach an idea is not a particularly *wabi-sabi* concept. It is, however, useful for this type of exploration, and, well, nothing is perfect.

3   There is, of course, a balance here. *Wabi-sabi* favors the non-perfect solution that we can accomplish, but it does not espouse sloppy actions or sub-standard results. For a deeper journey along an interesting side path looking at balancing structure and free-form elements of performance, consider the essay "Beat Zen, Square Zen, and Zen," by the philosopher Alan Watts. Watts, A. "Beat Zen, Square Zen, and Zen." http://www.thezensite.com/ZenEssays/Miscellaneous/Beat_Zen_Square_Zen.html.

07 | Understand Fallibility and Cognitive Bias

1   For a deeper review into the details of how cognitive biases function in general, an excellent and fascinating read is *Thinking, Fast and Slow* by Daniel Kahneman, the Nobel Prize-winning psychologist-economist who did some of the initial work identifying cognitive biases. Kahneman, D. *Thinking, Fast and Slow* (Farrar, Straus, and Grioux, 2011). Readers interested primarily in exploring the applications of cognitive biases might also enjoy the section on "Thinking Under Pressure," in Hearns, S. *Peak Performance Under Pressure: Lessons from a Helicopter Rescue Doctor* (Class Professional Publishing, 2019).

2   This phenomenon, often called base-rate neglect, is discussed extensively in Kahneman, D. *Thinking, Fast and Slow* (Farrar, Straus, and Grioux, 2011).

3   See for example, Gawande, A. *The Checklist Manifesto: How to Get Things Right* (Metropolitan Books, 2010).

08 | Become Comfortable with Uncertainty

1   Leschak, P. *Ghosts of the Fireground: Echoes of the Great Peshtigo Fire and the Calling of a Wildland Firefighter* (HarperOne, 2002).

2   The accuracy of a particular test (sodium or otherwise) for a particular patient is impacted by the characteristics of the test itself and how well the test applies to the patient at hand. The estimate of 1-2 mEq/L provided here is based on a conversation in 2013 with laboratory technicians at Massachusetts General Hospital in Boston, MA, whom I asked to estimate the error of the sodium measurements based on the methods they were using at the time. This might or might not be representative of the test error at a different hospital or at a different point in time. The reference laboratory at a hospital should be able to tell a provider the characteristics of a particular test at that hospital, which depends on the exact assay and equipment used. That said, the art of mapping the test to the patient is the responsibility of the provider, not the lab. Since the normal range of sodium is 135-145mEq/L, 1-2mEq/L is a small amount of variability.

3   Sometimes, as in the case of correcting sodium levels for hyperglycemia, there is a simple formula that allows us to mitigate the uncertainty of how a particular test result applies to a particular patient. See for example https://www.mdcalc.com/sodium-correction-hyperglycemia, which describes the classic equation correcting sodium measurements in this case. At other times, the relationship between the reported value and the ground truth is more complicated or might not be known.

4   Psychologist Kelly McGonigal, PhD has developed an arc of interesting and worthwhile experiments into how we can learn to choose our response to the physiological signals of stress. Her book, *The Upside of Stress*, is excellent. According to her data, merely considering the fact that you are able to choose part of your response to stress can yield significant benefits in performance under pressure. McGonical, K. *The Upside of Stress: Why Stress Is Good for You, and How to Get Good at It* (Avery, 2016).

09 | Harness the Wisdom of the Room

1   Duke, A. *Thinking in Bets: Making Smarter Decisions When You Don't Have All the Facts* (Portfolio, 2019).

2   I am deeply grateful to Dr. Chuck Pozner, Professor of Emergency Medicine at Harvard Medical School and the Medical Director of the Stratus Center for Medical Simulation, for teaching me and my teammates this mental framework, and reminding us of the importance of harnessing the wisdom of the room in difficult cases. I will admit that it might not always have seemed like I was grateful for the discussion at three o'clock in the morning, but I am.

3   See, for example, the section on "Decision Hygiene" in Duke, A. *How to Decide: Simple Tools for Making Better Choices* (Portfolio, 2020).

4   A great exploration of the differences between routine and critical communication, and how leaders can help guide the transitions between what is needed when comes from the Mission Critical Team Institute Podcast. Cline, P, and Ruiz, C. "Episode #2 Swarms, X-Teams, and Routine vs. Critical Communications" *MCTI Teamcast.* 2020. https://teamcast.missioncti.com/episode/2-swarms-x-teams-and-routine-vs-critical-communications.

10 | Make "Plan B" Part of the Plan

1   Dworkis, D. "Episode 16: Plan B is Part of the Plan," 2020, *The Emergency Mind Podcast.* https://soundcloud.com/emergencymind/episode-16.

2   For a deeper explanation of the Swiss cheese model and an exploration of other models of error, see Rutherford, G. "Introduction to Human Factors," in Rutherford, G. (Ed.), *Human Factors in Paramedic Practice* (Class Professional Publishing, 2020).

3   As our understanding of the risk of transmission of the COVID-19 virus grew, these initial triage plans were thankfully improved upon. Subsequent versions of the plan included objective methods of identifying potentially infected individuals, like temperature and oxygen saturation checks, as well as protocols for how to transition individuals from low-risk to high-risk areas as our knowledge about a patient evolved.

11 | Move from A to B to C

1   Like all algorithms, ABC has its limitations. For example, in some select circumstances, issues like the need to stop arterial bleeding (a circulation issue) may be more important than a breathing issue. In the vast majority of cases however, following the ABC algorithm provides patients with their best chance at survival.

2   For examples of algorithms supporting emergency performance at multiple levels, including algorithms that leverage hierarchies, see the section on "A Checklist for Checklists," in Hearns, S. *Peak Performance Under Pressure, Lessons From A Helicopter Rescue Doctor* (Class Professional Publishing, 2019).

3   An example of this from jiu-jitsu is the concept of "position before submission." Basically, this means that you need to establish the core

fundamentals that allow you to get to a hold or lock before attempting to finish it. As instructor Mark Mullen writes, "By all means, practice your submission skills, but understand that you can't submit unless you can GET TO your submission position!" Mullen, M. "Position Before Submission." https://graciebarra.com/gb-news/position-before-submission/.

12 | Learn to Ask Better Questions

1   On the topic of being preoccupied with what has already happened, as opposed to what we can do about it, the Stoic philosopher Seneca famously said, "Endeavor to never trip over something that is behind you." This is excellent advice both in and out of emergencies. I find saying it out loud to myself—"Dworkis, don't trip over something that's behind you,"—to be very helpful when I need to refocus on the present.

2   Authors Keller and Papasan ask a similarly structured question in their book *The ONE Thing*. Their question is, "What's the ONE Thing I can do such that by doing it everything else will be easier or unnecessary?" Keller, G. and Papasan, J. *The ONE Thing: The Surprisingly Simple Truth Behind Extraordinary Results* (Bard Press, 2013).

3   To be more specific, I actually told a brief version of the story of Dienekes and the Spartans who chose to stand and fight in the shade, as described in Chapter 20, Rapidly Accept Reality. Since we might be about to "fight in the shade" if the power went off completely, the team caught on quickly and easily refocused their attention to asking better questions.

13 | Eliminate Unnecessary Opportunities for Failure

1   Dworkis, D. "Episode 05: Eliminating Unnecessary Opportunities for Failure," 2019, *The Emergency Mind Podcast*. https://soundcloud.com/emergencymind/episode-5.

2   Dworkis, D. "Episode 25: Bridging the Why and the How," 2020, *The Emergency Mind Podcast*. https://soundcloud.com/emergencymind/episode-25.

3   See, for example, this article from author and Stoic Philosophy expert Ryan Holiday on the value of *premeditatio malorum*: Holiday, R. "The Surprising Value of Negative Thinking: A key to success that too few have figured out," *Psychology Today*, 2014. https://www.

psychologytoday.com/us/blog/the-obstacle-is-the-way/201405/ the-surprising-value-negative-thinking.

4   The idea of premortem thinking was first introduced by psychologist Gary Klein. See for example, Klein, G. *Sources of Power: How People Make Decisions* (MIT Press, 1999). Kahneman offers a great description of the premortem exercise here: https://www.youtube.com/ watch?v=MzTNMalfyhM.

14 | Decide to Not Decide

1   The juxtaposition of the decision logic between administering a thrombolytic and a CCB drip in acute stroke as presented here is a significant simplification. Depending on a variety of factors, either decision may be the more "important" one for a given patient. The relevant point is not how to treat acute strokes, but the fact that understanding the impact and relative "importance" of a particular decision is critical to optimizing efforts across a variety of decisions.

2   Former professional poker player turned decision-making expert Annie Duke talks extensively about freerolling in her book *How to Decide*. The chapter entitled "Breaking Free from Analysis Paralysis: How to Spend your Decision-Making Time More Wisely" should be required reading for anyone who performs under pressure. Duke, A. *How to Decide: Simple Tools for Making Better Choices* (Portfolio, 2020).

15 | Find the Rate-Limiting Step

1   See, for example, the following articles: "Rate Determining Step." 2020, https://chem.libretexts.org/@go/page/1412, or "Rate Determining Step," Illustrated Glossary of Organic Chemistry, http://www. chem.ucla.edu/~harding/IGOC/R/rate_determining_step.html.

2   I am simplifying this process slightly, since it is possible—though often less ideal—to use alternative pad configurations if a patient cannot be turned. Even when using these other approaches, generating an effective electrical current always requires two electrodes with the heart in the middle.

3   The concept of an emergency that is well-understood and mapped out might seem contradictory, but actually "routine emergencies" that can be planned for in advance do exist. As an interesting and worthwhile side path into this idea, consider reading Leonard, HB. and Howitt, AM. "High Performance in Emergency Preparedness and

Response: Disaster Type Differences" Taubman Center Policy Briefs, 2007. www.hks.harvard.edu/sites/default/files/centers/taubman/files/peril_new.pdf

16 | Commit to Never Waste Suffering

1   On the topic of making small improvements to your craft, consider this article by author James Clear on the accumulation of marginal gains: Clear, J, "This Coach Improved Every Tiny Thing by 1 Percent and Here's What Happened." https://jamesclear.com/marginal-gains

2   See, for example, this video on processing failure and learning in jiu-jitsu: Albin, N. "Losing is Learning in BJJ (IF you do it right)." https://www.youtube.com/watch?v=1sVXVR72h0k&t=2s.

3   The Harvard T.H. Chan School of Public Health offers an excellent introduction to root cause analyses in this video: "How To Conduct a Root Cause Analysis of a Critical Incident." https://www.youtube.com/watch?v=iIis4YloV8Q.

4   The first time I wrote this sentence, I ended it with "*or* in five years." Changing it to "*and*" in five years opens up a further line of thought: when you're doing an analysis about how to leverage suffering into structural improvements, what happens when you take a long-term view like this and envision solutions that are designed to last years? Since emergency residency training is four years, a solution that works tomorrow, the next day, and in five years requires building something that outlasts the institutional memory of any one trainee.

5   See, for example, the paper on the concept of "residue" from the folks at the Mission Critical Teams Institute: Cline, P, "Residue," Mission Critical Teams Institute. https://missioncti.com/wp-content/uploads/2020/06/RESIDUE-V.4-PUBLIC-DISTRIBUTION-4.20.20-1.pdf.

17 | Humans Not Robots

1   Dworkis, D. "Episode 18: Bringing Your Whole Self to Work", 2020, *The Emergency Mind Podcast*. https://soundcloud.com/emergency-mind/episode-18.

2   See, for example: Mildenhall, J. "Well-Being of the Paramedic," Rutherford, G. (Ed.), *Human Factors in Paramedic Medicine* (Class Professional Publishing, 2020).

3   U.S. Department of Transportation, Federal Aviation Administration, Flight Standards Service. *Risk Management Handbook*, 2009, Change 1

(January 2016). www.faa.gov/regulations_policies/handbooks_manuals/aviation/media/risk_management_hb_change_1.pdf

4   Cline, P. "Residue," Mission Critical Teams Institute, 2020. https://missioncti.com/wp-content/uploads/2020/06/RESIDUE-V.4-PUBLIC-DISTRIBUTION-4.20.20-1.pdf.

5   Dworkis, D. "Episode 24: Performance is a Choice," 2020, *The Emergency Mind Podcast.* https://soundcloud.com/emergencymind/episode-24.

18 | Start From First Principles

1   See for example this collection of ethics-based cases in emergency medicine from the Society of Academic Emergency Medicine: Dancour, EE. "Ethical Issues in Emergency Medicine." https://www.saem.org/cdem/education/online-education/m3-curriculum/professionalism/ethical-issues-in-the-ed.

2   See for example, the START triage system from the US Department of Health and Human Services. https://chemm.nlm.nih.gov/startadult.htm#more.

3   The American College of Emergency Physicians, for example, provides guidance on a "code of ethics" covering a variety of issues ranging from end-of-life care to social media use. https://www.acep.org/patient-care/policy-statements/code-of-ethics-for-emergency-physicians/.

19 | Favor Praxis Over Theory

1   Lovell, JA. "Apollo Expeditions to the Moon 13.4." https://history.nasa.gov/SP-350/ch-13-4.html.

2   Reimer, B. "NASA 'Hacks:' The Real Stories," 2015. https://www.nasa.gov/feature/nasa-hacks-the-real-stories .

3   For detailed accounts of helicopter transport missions and the thought that goes into them, see the section on "Pressure Management Case Studies" in Hearns, S. *Peak Performance Under Pressure: Lessons from a Helicopter Rescue Doctor* (Class Professional Publishing, 2019).

4   On the subject of sharing knowledge about what works on the ground with all parts of an organization, authors Lobdell et al describe a useful tool called a "fusion cell," which brings individuals with theoretical knowledge to the same table with individuals with practical knowledge to facilitate decision making. Lobdell, KW et al. "Improving

Health Care Leadership in the Covid-19 Era." *NEJM Catal*, 2020. https://catalyst.nejm.org/doi/full/10.1056/CAT.20.0225.

5   A useful way to think systematically about the differences between what it takes logistically to deliver these two doses of vancomycin is to compare the concepts of work-as-done and work-as-imagined. Essentially, work-as-done describes what actually happens on the ground, whereas work-as-imagined describes how things are supposed to function in theory. See, for example, McNab, D. and Rutherford, G. "Systems Thinking," in Rutherford, G. (Ed), *Human Factors in Paramedic Practice* (Class Professional Publishing, 2020).

20 | Rapidly Accept Reality

1   This story is sometimes attributed to the Spartan king, Leonidas I.

2   See for example the recommendations from the Canadian Airway Focus Group, which summarized and reviewed multiple large case registries on difficult airway management (Law, JA. et al. "The difficult airway with recommendations for management—Part 1—Difficult tracheal intubation encountered in an unconscious/induced patient," *Can J Anaesth* 2013 Nov;60(11):1089-118). The Japanese Emergency Medicine Network Investigators also found evidence of the importance of moving early in airway management from routine to rescue protocols. (Goto, T. et al, "Multiple failed intubation attempts are associated with decreased success rates on the first rescue intubation in the emergency department: a retrospective analysis of multicentre observational data." *Scand J Trauma Resusc Emerg Med* 2015 Jan 16;23:5.)

3   Gonzales, L. *Deep Survival: Who Lives, Who Dies, and Why* (W.W. Norton and Company, 2013, 2017).

4   This is an example both of anchoring bias and of confirmation bias, as described more in Chapter 7, Understand Fallibility and Cognitive Bias.

21 | See the Forest and the Leaf

1   For the details of this regulation, which are interesting and worth a read, see: Flight Crewmember Duties 14 CFR §121.542 (1981).

2   For a more emergency-specific contextualization of the Flight Crewmember Duties regulation, see Lauria, M. "COMM CHECK: Sterile Cockpit." *EMCrit Blog*, 2018. https://emcrit.org/emcrit/comm-check-sterile-cockpit/.

3   Gray SH, Lauria MJ, and Hicks C. "The Mindset of the Resuscitationist," *Emerg. Med. Clin. N. Am.* 2020, 38(4):739-753.

4   For more examples of helpful exercises for consciously altering the scope of your focus during a crisis, see the excellent section on "Concentration Skills and Mental Toughness," in Asken, MJ., Grossman, D., and Christensen, LW. *Warrior Mindset: Mental Toughness Skills for a Nation's Peacekeepers.* (Human Factor Research Group, 2010).

22 | Find Your Locus of Control

1   Epictetus. *The Enchiridion.* Carter, E. (Trans.) http://classics.mit.edu/Epictetus/epicench.html.

2   In their book on leadership and management, The ONE Thing, Gary Keller and Jay Papasan ask a similarly structured question designed to help focus your energy where you have the most control. Their version of the question is "What's the ONE Thing I can do such that by doing it everything else will be easier or unnecessary?" Keller, G. and Papasan, J. *The ONE Thing: The Surprisingly Simple Truth Behind Extraordinary Results* (Bard Press, 2013).

3   Duke, A. *Thinking in Bets: Making Smarter Decisions When You Don't Have All the Facts* (Portfolio, 2019).

4   Neuroscientist Andrew Huberman, PhD, does a great job breaking down the science of how breathing influences our response to stress in his podcast. Huberman, A. "Episode 10: Master Stress: Tools for Managing Stress & Anxiety," 2021, *Huberman Lab.* https://huberman-lab.libsyn.com/master-stress-tools-for-managing-stress-anxiety-epi-sode-10.

23 | Treat the Individuals and the Field

1   Antonsen, E. Personal communication, paraphrased. 2013.

2   Groups of individuals who assemble rapidly to address unplanned events like code-blue activations are sometimes called "swarm" teams. Participating in or leading a swarm team is a unique challenge, as often the team members have never worked together and may have vastly different training experiences. If you are likely to be a member of this kind of team, I highly recommend the Mission Critical Teams Institute briefing on swarm teams. https://teamcast.missioncti.com/episode/2-swarms-x-teams-and-routine-vs-critical-communications.

3   See, for example, the "Take Action" section of Chapter 01 Find the Calm in the Storm.

24 | Combine Action and Analysis

1   In cases when you need to intervene but do not have a clear mental picture of the underlying situation, algorithmic thinking, like the ABC approach discussed in Chapter 11, Move from A to B to C, can be particularly helpful.

2   A great example of training immediate action around hemorrhage control is the STOP THE BLEED campaign. www.Stopthebleed.org.

3   Identifying patterns in data that suggest an impending crisis is a deeply important and fascinating skill that relies on expertise, training, and practice. For more on how experienced operators use this ability, see the section on "The Power to See the Invisible" in Klein, G. *Sources of Power: How People Make Decisions* (The MIT Press, 1999).

4   In the setting of a cervical-spine injury or instability, the head tilt is contraindicated, and the relevant provider would have to be more thoughtful on their initial approach.

5   As an important corollary to this, do not run in the emergency department unless there is a really good reason to.

6   See, for example, the "Jerk and Check" episode of the EMCrit Podcast. Weingart, S. "EMCrit 293 – The Jerk & Check, Functional Heuristics in Resuscitation Project (MotR)." *EMCrit Blog,* 2021. https://emcrit.org/emcrit/functional-heuristics-in-resuscitation/.

25 | Use Algorithmic and Creative Thinking

1   See, for example, Nickson, C. "Post-intubation hypoxia," 2015, *Life in the Fast Lane Blog.* //litfl.com/post-intubation-hypoxia/.

2   For a deeper dive into how experts generate and mentally test potential solutions to a particular problem, see the section on "The Power of Mental Simulation," in Klein, G. *Sources of Power: How People Make Decisions* (The MIT Press, 1999). Klein's work suggests that experts do not generate a set of options and compare between them, but instead, move serially through options, mentally testing each one as they go.

3   Dworkis, D. "Episode 14: Standby for Chaos," 2020, *The Emergency Mind Podcast.* https://soundcloud.com/emergencymind/episode-14.

4   Hearns, S. *Peak Performance Under Pressure: Lessons from a Helicopter Rescue Doctor* (Class Professional Publishing, 2019).

5   See, for example, the section on "The Power of Intuition," in Klein, G. *Sources of Power: How People Make Decisions* (The MIT Press, 1999).

6   An excellent and worthwhile read exploring creative problem solving at sea is Callahan, S. *Adrift: Seventy-Six Days Lost at Sea* (Mariner Books, 2002).

7   Dworkis, D. "Episode 07: Algorithms and Jazz," 2019, *The Emergency Mind Podcast*. https://soundcloud.com/emergencymind/episode-7.

8   Gawande, A. *The Checklist Manifesto: How to Get Things Right* (Metropolitan Books, 2010).

9   This is somewhat of a simplification, as more complex algorithms can and do incorporate external inputs, link to other algorithms, or involve probabilistic reasoning that could yield a variety of types of solutions.

Printed in the USA
CPSIA information can be obtained
at www.ICGtesting.com
LVHW041528221123
764628LV00004B/304